COVID's Impact on Health and Healthcare Workers

T0073724

COVID's Impact on Health and Healthcare Workers

Don L. Goldenberg, MD

Emeritus Professor of Medicine, Tufts University School of Medicine
Adjunct Faculty, Departments of Medicine & Nursing,
Oregon Health Sciences University

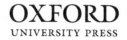

OXFORD
UNIVERSITY PRESS

Oxford University Press is a department of the University of Oxford. It furthers
the University's objective of excellence in research, scholarship, and education
by publishing worldwide. Oxford is a registered trade mark of Oxford University
Press in the UK and certain other countries.

Published in the United States of America by Oxford University Press
198 Madison Avenue, New York, NY 10016, United States of America.

© Oxford University Press 2021

Library of Congress Cataloging-in-Publication Data
Names: Goldenberg, Don L., author.
Title: COVID's impact on health and healthcare workers / Don L. Goldenberg.
Description: New York, NY : Oxford University Press, [2021] |
Includes bibliographical references and index. |
Identifiers: LCCN 2021006872 (print) | LCCN 2021006873 (ebook) |
ISBN 9780197575390 (paperback) | ISBN 9780197575413 (epub) | ISBN 9780197575420
Subjects: MESH: COVID-19 | Hospitalization | Health Personnel | Pandemics |
Health Services | Delivery of Health Care | United States
Classification: LCC RA644.C67 (print) | LCC RA644.C67 (ebook) |
NLM WC 506 | DDC 616.2/414—dc23
LC record available at https://lccn.loc.gov/2021006872
LC ebook record available at https://lccn.loc.gov/2021006873

DOI: 10.1093/med/9780197575390.001.0001

1 3 5 7 9 8 6 4 2

Printed by LSC communications, United States of America

This book is dedicated to the countless heroic healthcare workers who have toiled through the worst health crisis in a century.

Contents

Acknowledgments

I am grateful for everyone at Oxford University Press, most importantly Andrea Knobloch and Jacqueline Buckley, for their thoughts and assistance. Dr. Howard Ory and Dr. Marc Dichter were kind enough to review drafts of the book and provide important suggestions. As always, my wife, Patty, encouraged and supported me, as we hunkered down side by side in this difficult year.

Introduction

When I began this book a year ago, my objective was to provide a comprehensive summary of how the COVID-19 pandemic had affected our health and our healthcare professionals. As the pandemic surged on, I had to revise this goal. It quickly became apparent that "comprehensive" was unrealistic. In March 2020, I began reviewing each new medical article on COVID-19, but through May 31, the last day I tried to keep up, 4,500 peer-reviewed papers dedicated to the pandemic had already been published. It became obvious that I would need to become more selective. Currently, there are more than 65,000 scientific articles under the search term "coronavirus/covid-19" that pop up on PubMed.

Since my interest and expertise are in clinical medicine, I have focused on those aspects of the pandemic that have been of the greatest clinical relevance to patients and to their healthcare providers. This book does not delve into pathophysiology, genetics, transmission, diagnostic tests, and epidemiology. Because targeted treatments had only a modest impact on the pandemic, I limited discussion about specific COVID-19 therapies. Rather than review the pandemic's global healthcare impact, I focused on what has transpired in the United States, with a selected review of the pandemic's healthcare impact in the United Kingdom and a few other countries.

My second objective, to provide the reader with a summary on how the pandemic played out, also needed to be rethought. COVID-19 was raging on just as strongly on February 1, 2021, as on that date 1 year ago. At that time, no one would have predicted that things would still be so bleak. There had been a number of coronavirus epidemics in the previous decade, but they had been largely contained within a few months. China, the initial COVID-19 epicenter, had essentially eradicated its cases in early 2020 with aggressive shutdowns and massive testing and tracing. Back in January, the virus genome had been sequenced and in a matter of weeks that information allowed scientists to begin the development of an effective vaccine. Hundreds of clinical trials were being done throughout the world with a vast array of medications and novel therapeutics. Yet, 1 year later, our health was still at risk and our healthcare workers still struggled mightily to combat the pandemic. So rather than just looking back, I have endeavored to also look ahead. In each chapter, I selectively reviewed the most essential studies from key medical reports and inserted first-hand descriptions and explanations from various media sources. Chapter 1 focuses on the symptoms and typical course of COVID-19 infections, from mild/moderate to severe. It explores fluctuations in hospitalizations and mortality during the pandemic as well as the adverse impact of the pandemic on non-COVID urgent medical conditions. The next chapter reviews the individual risk factors for COVID infection and disease severity, including patient age, comorbidities such as obesity and diabetes, residence in long-term care facilities, gender, and race/ethnicity. Chapter 3 provides a detailed evaluation of the impact of the pandemic on healthcare workers and on hospitals. The next two chapters focus on the major changes in primary care and specialty practices as a result of the pandemic, including the expansion of telemedicine. Chapter 6 highlights the negative impact of misinformation and disinformation during the pandemic. The following chapter focuses on persistent medical problems, long after the initial COVID infection, including potential organ damage and multiple, unexplained symptoms. This chapter also explores the potential mental health fallout in the general population. Finally, I recommend some approaches to aid our pandemic recovery and to help prevent similar future disasters: make public health a national priority, erase healthcare inequities, improve care of the elderly and long-term care facilities, shore up primary care, ensure the well-being of our healthcare workers, and foster public confidence in science.

Early in my career, I was interested in the relationship of infectious agents to rheumatic diseases, and no infectious disease has been as challenging as COVID-19. Subsequently, I dedicated much of my practice and research to fibromyalgia, chronic fatigue syndrome, and overlapping illness. This background meshed with the recent growing attention to the prolonged symptoms in millions of patients following COVID-19 infection.

After retiring from practice 5 years ago and moving to Portland, Oregon, I have continued to stay involved in clinical research and teaching in my role as Emeritus Professor of Medicine at Tufts University School of Medicine and adjunct faculty member in the Departments of Medicine and Nursing at Oregon Health Sciences University. I have had the opportunity to stay current and to review important medical literature as an author and section editor for *UptoDate*. During the past year I became the section editor for the new topic, Coronavirus disease 2019 (COVID-19): Care of patients with systemic rheumatic disease during the pandemic. Being retired from the practice of medicine has provided me with the time to pursue this book project. The shelter-in-place isolation during the past year afforded me countless hours each day to digest the reams of medical articles pouring out.

As I finish this book, the COVID-19 pandemic has reached an inflection point. With effective vaccines we can picture an end to its constant threat. Yet much of the world is mired in persistent danger. Looking back on what has transpired during the pandemic provides important lessons for our nation's recovery and can guide us in preparing better for the future.

. . . *and then the ending of the plague became the target of all hopes. We should go forward, groping our way through the darkness, stumbling perhaps at times, and try to do what good lay in our power.*

—Albert Camus, *The Plague* (1947)

1

COVID-19 Infection

Mild and Moderate COVID-19

More than 80% of documented COVID-19 infections have been considered mild to moderate.[1] This doesn't include asymptomatic cases, which account for 40%–50% of all cases.[2]

Knowing that one is an asymptomatic carrier has its own set of concerns, as Dr. Rucha Mehta Shah learned: "Little did I know that—while certainly not as traumatic as falling ill—living asymptomatically with coronavirus in the United States would come with its own horrors. When I got the call that I had tested positive, I froze. I had so many questions but could not vocalize any of them. While I am lucky not to have experienced symptoms, asymptomatic disease is still disease. The symptoms are just hidden: feelings of guilt, isolation, fear of infecting those you love, fear of potentially getting sicker."[3]

The most common presenting symptoms in patients with COVID infection are fever, cough, fatigue, and dyspnea (Figure 1.1).[4] Typical COVID symptoms have been much more alarming than seasonal flu. Different patients reported, "I woke up with a headache that was Top 5 of my life, like someone inside my head was trying to push my eyes out. I got a 100.6-degree fever . . . Everything hurt. Nothing in my body felt like it was working. I felt so beat up, like I had been in a boxing ring with Mike Tyson. I had a fever and chills—one minute my teeth are chattering and the next minute I am sweating like I am in a sauna. And the heavy, hoarse cough, my God. The

[1] CDC COVID Data Tracker. Coronavirus Disease 2019. April 20, 2020.

[2] Oran DP, Topol EJ. Prevalence of asymptomatic SARS-CoV-2 infection. *Ann Intern Med*. September 1, 2020. https://doi.org/10.7326/M20-3012.

[3] Shah RM. The horror of living with coronavirus asymptomatically. *The Washington Post*. July 21, 2020.

[4] Sheleme T, Bekele F, Ayela T. Clinical presentation of patients infected with coronavirus disease 19: A systematic review. *Infect Dis (Auckl)*. September 10, 2020. doi: 10.1177/1178633720952076.

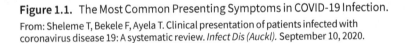

Figure 1.1. The Most Common Presenting Symptoms in COVID-19 Infection.

From: Sheleme T, Bekele F, Ayela T. Clinical presentation of patients infected with coronavirus disease 19: A systematic review. *Infect Dis (Auckl).* September 10, 2020.

cough rattled through my whole body. You know how a car sounds when the engine is puttering? That is what it sounded like . . . On Day 10, I woke up at 2:30 a.m. holding a pillow on my chest. I felt like there was an anvil sitting on my chest. Not a pain, not any kind of jabbing—just very heavy . . . It was just a loss of all energy and drive. There was no horizontal surface in my house that I didn't want to just lay down on all day long."[5]

Reduction of smell, anosmia, has been one of the most predictive early symptoms since it is uncommon in other viral respiratory infections but present in 20%–70% of COVID-19 cases.[6] Smell and taste dysfunction have been especially prominent in younger, nonhospitalized patients. Among

[5] Burch ADS, Cargill C, Frankenfield J, Harmon A, Robertson C, Sinha S, et al. "An anvil sitting on my chest": What it's like to have Covid-19. *The New York Times.* May 6, 2020.

[6] Tong JY, Wong A, Zhu D, Fastenberg JH, Tham T. The prevalence of olfactory and gustatory dysfunction in COVID-19 patients: A systematic review and meta-analysis. *Otolaryngol Head Neck Surg.* 2020;163(1):3–11. doi: 10.1177/0194599820926473.

567 adults who reported a loss of taste or smell in the prior month, 77% tested positive for SARS-CoV-2 antibodies.[7] Loss of both smell and taste was more strongly associated with antibody positivity than loss of taste alone. Dr. Tim Spector, one of the investigators in the COVID Symptom Study, noted that it took a few months for clinicians to recognize the diagnostic importance of anosmia, which was 10 times more predictive of COVID than any other single symptom.[8]

A wide variety of gastrointestinal and dermatologic symptoms were also reported. In data from the COVID Symptom Study, 17% of patients said they had experienced a rash.[9] The rashes included hives; a diffuse papular, erythematous eruption; and reddish/purplish bumps on the fingers or toes, termed "COVID toes." In 20% of cases, the rash was the only presenting symptom. COVID fingers and toes has been the most characteristic rash associated with COVID infection and has been reported in as many as 40% of cases.[10]

Symptoms have varied with age, disease severity, and underlying health. Dr. Mark A. Perazella, professor of medicine at Yale School of Medicine, noted, "The problem is that it depends on who you are and how healthy you are. It's so heterogeneous, it's hard to say. If you're healthy, most likely you'll get fever, achiness, nasal symptoms, dry cough, and you'll feel crappy. But there are going to be the oddballs that are challenging and come in with some symptoms and nothing else, and you don't suspect Covid."[11]

COVID symptoms were very unpredictable, as Robert Baird, a writer for *The New Yorker*, described in his own illness, "One of the strange and unsettling features of covid-19, as a disease, is that it appears to progress in a nonlinear fashion: people often feel bad, and then better, and then bad again.

[7] Makaronidis J, Mok J, Balogun N, Magee CG, Omar RZ, Carnemolla A. Seroprevalence of SARS-CoV-2 antibodies in people with an acute loss in their sense of smell and/or taste in a community-based population in London, UK: An observational cohort study. *PLoS Med.* October 1, 2020. https://doi.org/10.1371/journal.pmed.1003358.

[8] Menni C, Sudre CH, Steves CJ, Ourselin S, Spector TD. Quantifying additional COVID-19 symptoms will save lives. *Lancet.* 2020 Jun 20;395(10241):e107–e108.

[9] Menni C, Valdes AM, Freidin MB, Sudre CH, Nguyen LH, Drew DA, et al. Real-time tracking of self-reported symptoms to predict potential of COVID-19. *Nature Medicine.* 2020;26:1037–1040.

[10] Daneshgaran G, Dubin DP, Gould DJ. Cutaneous manifestations of COVID-19: An evidence-based review. *Am J Clin Dermatol.* 2020;21:627–639. doi:10.1007/s40257-020-00558-4.

[11] Parker-Pope T. The many symptoms of Covid-19. *The New York Times.* August 5, 2020. Accessed August 5, 2020. https://www.newyorktimes.com/

The possibility of a sudden downturn, it seems, is one that can't be dismissed until you recover completely."[12]

Mild to moderate COVID infection has generally been classified as one not requiring hospital admission. Over time it became clear that the duration of symptoms, even in mild to moderate COVID, was often longer than the 7–10 days reported in early studies. More than 90% of outpatients reported persistent symptoms 2–3 weeks after an initial positive test for COVID-19.[13] Fever had resolved in 97%, but cough had not resolved in 43% and fatigue was still present in 35%. One-third of these patients initially reported dyspnea, and one-third of those were still short of breath at 2–3 weeks. One-quarter of those aged 18–34 years and one-half of those aged >50 years had not returned to their previous health at the 2–3-week interview.

The severity of pulmonary symptoms has been the most important factor in predicting disease severity. The initial public health advice was to stay at home unless you developed severe breathing difficulty. It wasn't until later that we recognized how quickly and silently COVID pneumonia progressed. Dr. Richard Levitan, an emergency room physician, noted, "From a public health perspective, we've been wrong to tell people to come back only if they have severe shortness of breath. Toughing it out is not a great strategy."[14] In most hospitalized patients, shortness of breath did not develop until a median of 5–8 days after symptom onset. Dr. Leora Horwitz, associate professor of medicine at NYU, advised: "With Covid, I tell people that around a week is when I want you to really pay attention to how you're feeling. Don't get complacent and feel like it's all over."[15] Dr. Charles A. Powell, director of the Mount Sinai-National Jewish Health Respiratory Institute, advised: "The major thing we worry about is a worsening at eight to 12 days—an increasing shortness of breath, worsening cough."[16]

---

[12] Baird RP. How doctors on the front lines are confronting the uncertainties of COVID-19. *The New Yorker*. April 5, 2020. Accessed October 9, 2020. https://newyorker.com

[13] Tenforde MW, Kim SS, Lindsell CJ, Rose EB, Shapiro NI, Files DC, et al. Symptom duration and risk factors for delayed return to usual health among outpatients with COVID-19 in a multistate health care systems network—United States, March–June 2020. *MMWR*. 2020 Jul 31;69(30):993–998.

[14] Levitan R. The infection that's silently killing coronavirus patients. *The New York Times*. April 20, 2020. Accessed May 1, 2020. https://www.newyorktimes.com/

[15] Parker-Pope T. The many symptoms of Covid-19. *The New York Times*. August 8, 2020. Accessed September 2, 2020. https://www.newyorktimes.com/

[16] Parker-Pope T. The many symptoms of Covid-19. *The New York Times*. August 8, 2020. Accessed September 2, 2020. https://www.newyorktimes.com/

It has been very difficult to determine whether any medications decrease the risk of severe COVID or hospitalization. There is evidence that monoclonal antibodies decrease the risk of severe COVID-19 and keep patients out of the hospital, but they have not been widely prescribed. As of January 1, 2021, less than 20% of the federal supply of monoclonal antibodies had been used at hospitals in the United States.[17,18] One relatively small study found that early administration of high-titer convalescent plasma against SARS-CoV-2 to mildly infected older patients reduced the risk of progression to severe respiratory disease.[19]

Dr. Janet Shapiro described her recurrent symptoms after recovering from what she thought was a mild COVID-19 infection: "However, after a few days, I felt worse, sensing that my heart rate was going fast even when I woke up. But I could not maintain the pace in the hospital, I could not breathe with my N95, I could not even stand for rounds. I was sent home to monitor my vital signs and with the instruction to rest and avoid stress, an impossible prescription for these times. The symptoms of chest tightness gradually subsided and, fortunately, the echocardiogram and laboratory parameters improved. What were the lessons of a relatively mild case for this physician-patient? COVID-19 is really, really tragic, worse than we could have ever expected. I experienced what it is to feel one's body, the difficulty of a breath, a fast heartbeat, the vagueness of feeling unwell and the fear it brings. This is what patients experience on a daily basis. No one is safe from illness."[20]

Severe Infection, Hospitalization, and Death

During the early phases of the pandemic, approximately 5% of patients with COVID-19 infection developed severe symptoms, requiring hospitalization, with about one-third immediately admitted to an intensive care unit (ICU).[21]

[17] McGinley L. Only one covid-19 treatment is designed to keep people out of the hospital. Many overburdened hospitals are not offering it. *The Washington Post*. December 31, 2020.

[18] McGinley, L. Only one covid-19 treatment is designed to keep people out of the hospital. Many overburdened hospitals are not offering it. *The Washington Post*. December 31, 2020.

[19] Libster R, Perez Marc G, Wappner D, Coviello S, Bianchi A, Braem V, et al. Early high-titer plasma therapy to prevent severe Covid-19 in older adults. *N Engl J Med*. January 6, 2020. doi: 10.1056/NEJMoa2033700. https://www.nejm.org/doi/full/10.1056/NEJMoa2033700

[20] Shapiro JM. Having coronavirus disease 2019 (COVID-19). *JAMA Cardiol*. 2020;5:1091. doi: 10.1001/jamacardio.2020.3247.

[21] Wu Z, McGoogan JM. Characteristics of and important lessons from the coronavirus disease 2019 (COVID-19) outbreak in China: Summary of a report of 72 314 cases from the

The average interval of onset of symptoms to hospitalization was 7 days,[22] and more than 80% of patients were hospitalized directly from home.[23]

Dr. Danielle Ofri described the alarming features of one of her first critically ill COVID-19 patients at Bellevue Hospital. "She's already intubated, sedated, and paralyzed, but her temperature has started to jump the rails: first it's 103.8, then 104.5, then 105.3. Three of us gingerly roll her to one side and attempt to slide an electric cooling blanket beneath her, without dislodging her breathing tube, arterial line, cardiac monitors, or I.V. drips. Her temperature hits 106.1. We cram specimen bags with ice as quickly as we can, tucking them into her armpits, under her neck, and between her legs. They turn to water almost on contact. Her temperature is now 106.9, and her pulse has soared to a hundred and seventy."[24]

The mortality rate in hospitalized patients during the early months of the pandemic was 20%–30%. In Lombardy, Italy, 88% of hospitalized patients required mechanical ventilation and more than a quarter of the patients died.[25] Of the 5,700 patients hospitalized in New York, 14% were treated in the ICU, 12% received mechanical ventilation, and 21% died.[26] Almost 90% of patients who received mechanical ventilation died. In an early UK study of more than 20,000 hospitalized COVID-19 patients, 26% had died and another 34% were still receiving in-hospital care at the end of data collection.[27] In another series of 1,000 hospitalized patients in New York,

Chinese Center for Disease Control and Prevention. *JAMA*. February 24, 2020. 2020 Apr 7;323:1239–1242.

[22] Garg S, Kim L, Whitaker M, O'Halloran A, Cummings C, Holstein R, et al. Hospitalization rates and characteristics of patients hospitalized with laboratory-confirmed coronavirus disease 2019—COVID-NET, 14 States, March 1–30, 2020. *MMWR*. 2020;69:458–464.

[23] Lavery AM, Preston LE, Ko JY, Chevinsky JR, DeSisto CL, Pennington AF, et al. Characteristics of hospitalized COVID-19 patients discharged and experiencing same-hospital readmission–United States, March–August 2020. *MMWR*. 2020;69:1695–1699.

[24] Ofri D. A Bellevue doctor's pandemic diary. *The New Yorker*. October 1, 2020.

[25] Grasselli G, Zangrillo A, Zanella A, Antonelli M, Cabrini L, Castelli A, et al. Baseline characteristics and outcomes of 1591 patients infected with SARS-CoV-2 admitted to ICUs of the Lombardy region, Italy. *JAMA*. 2020;323(16):1574–1581. April 6, 2020. doi:10.1001/jama.2020.5394.

[26] Richardson S, Hirsch JS, Narasimhan M, Crawford JM, McGinn T, Davidson KW, et al. Presenting characteristics, comorbidities, and outcomes among 5700 patients hospitalized with COVID-19 in the New York City area. *JAMA*. 2020;323(20):2052–2059. Apr 22. 10.1001/jama.2020.6775.

[27] Docherty AB, Harrison EM, Green CA, Hardwick HE, Pius R, Norman L, et al. Features of 20 133 UK patients in hospital with covid-19 using the ISARIC WHO Clinical Characterisation Protocol: Prospective observational cohort study. *BMJ*. 2020;369:m1985.

acute respiratory distress occurred in 35%, including 90% in the ICU, acute kidney injury in 34%, with 13% requiring dialysis, and new-onset cardiac arrhythmia in 9%.[28] A systematic review of 25,000 patients from various countries with severe coronavirus disease found that 32% of patients with COVID-19 were admitted to the ICU and the mortality in those patients was 39% during the first few months of the pandemic.[29]

Dr. Christopher Chen described his own case of severe COVID-19 while hospitalized in the ICU as being "like dying in solitary confinement." He continued: "Nights were the worst. That's when the fevers were highest and my breathing was most labored. I felt like I was wasting away: covered in sweat, unable to bathe or shower, tied down by a web of wires, lines, and tubes and trying desperately to breathe. I got an inkling of what my heart failure patients experience when they cannot breathe due to fluid buildup in their lungs and feel like they are drowning from the inside out."[30]

Dr. Levitan said, "Even patients without respiratory complaints had Covid pneumonia. When Covid pneumonia first strikes, patients don't feel short of breath, even as their oxygen levels fall. And by the time they do, they have alarmingly low oxygen levels and moderate-to-severe pneumonia (as seen on chest X-rays). To my amazement, most patients I saw said they had been sick for a week or so with fever, cough, upset stomach, and fatigue, but they only became short of breath the day they came to the hospital. Their pneumonia had clearly been going on for days, but by the time they felt they had to go to the hospital, they were often already in critical condition."[31] At that stage patients often can't maintain adequate oxygen supply and need to be intubated. As described by Dr. Dhruv Khullar, "A tube is snaked down a patient's throat and into the lungs. All intubated patients are transferred to an I.C.U. The ventilator takes over the work of breathing; doctors treat what they can and hope for the best."[32]

[28] Argenziano MG, Bruce SL, Slater CL, Tiao JR, Baldwin MR, Barr RG, et al. Characterization and clinical course of 1000 patients with coronavirus disease 2019 in New York; retrospective case series. *BMJ.* 2020;369:m1996. doi: 10.1136/bmj.m1996.

[29] Abate SM, Ale SA, Mantfardo B, Basu B. Rate of intensive care unit admission and outcomes among patients with coronavirus: A systematic review and meta-analysis. *PLoS One.* 2020 Jul 10;15(7):e0235653.

[30] Chen C. My severe Covid-19: It felt like dying in solitary confinement. *STAT.* August 28, 2020.

[31] Levitan R. The infection that's silently killing coronavirus patients. *The New York Times.* April 20, 2020. Accessed April 22, 2020. https://www.newyorktimes.com/

[32] Khullar D. How to understand Trump's evolving condition. *The New Yorker.* October 4, 2020. https://newyorker.com

Dr. Clayton Dalton, at Massachusetts General Hospital, described the downhill trajectory of COVID patients requiring intubation: "Ultimately, the ventilator is not a cure for covid-19; the machine can only provide support while doctors monitor and hope for improvement. Other patients continue to deteriorate, or perhaps just plateau with no sign of improvement, and so the I.C.U. team and family members must make a difficult decision about when to transition to end-of life care. There used to be a designated room for those conversations, adjacent to the unit, but now they take place on the telephone, or through Zoom or FaceTime. Once it's agreed that further treatment is likely to be futile, the team shifts to comfort measures. Dialysis machines are powered down; I.V. pumps are disconnected; the vitals monitor is turned off, and its colored numbers disappear. Alarms go quiet, and the room falls silent. Morphine is given to ease pain and air hunger. Other medications decrease respiratory secretions, so that breathing can be as unencumbered as possible. Finally, the tube is removed, as delicately as possible, and the patient takes his or her last breaths."[33]

As Dr. Clayton noted, most critically ill patients during the early stages of the pandemic were treated with mechanical ventilation. Subsequently, there was a greater focus on postponing mechanical ventilation and avoiding it altogether when possible. Moving patients onto their stomachs, so-called awake proning, was helpful, but not easy. "During the pandemic, proning has been shown to make a lifesaving difference for some patients; it allows the fluid in the lungs to redistribute itself, opening up new areas to oxygenation. But carefully flipping an unconscious, paralyzed patient can require as many as six people—nurses, assistants, therapists, and sometimes doctors, each gowned in P.P.E.—to coordinate their efforts, as though they are moving a large sculpture. In order for an I.C.U. to prone large numbers of patients each day, it must be fully staffed."[34] Awake proning and relative safety of high-flow nasal cannula oxygen have provided effective alternatives to mechanical ventilation.[35]

Large, university medical centers with ample critical care staff, equipment, and facilities were most capable of handling the sickest patients. In a study of 2,215 adults admitted to ICUs across the United States from March 4 to

---

[33] Dalton C. The risks of normalizing the coronavirus. *The New Yorker*. May 27, 2020.

[34] Nuila R. To fight the coronavirus, you need an army. *The New Yorker*. July 17, 2020.

[35] Bos LDJ, Brodie D, Calfee SC. Severe COVID-19 infections: Knowledge gained and remaining questions. *JAMA Intern Med*. 2021 Jan 1;181(1):9–11.

April 4, 2020, COVID-infected patients admitted to hospitals with fewer than 50 ICU beds had a threefold higher risk of death than those admitted to hospitals with more than 100 ICU beds.[36] Dr. Daniela Lamas recounted the importance of expert hospital critical care: "While even the best possible treatment couldn't save everyone, those who survived did so because of meticulous critical care, which requires a combination of resources and competency that is only available to a minority of hospitals in this country. And now, even as we race toward the hope of a magic bullet for this virus, we must openly acknowledge that disparity—and work to address it . . . we must also devote resources to helping hospitals deliver high-quality critical care. Maybe that will mean better allocating the resources we do have through a more robust, coordinated system of hospital-to-hospital patient transfers within each region. Maybe it means creating something akin to dedicated coronavirus centers of excellence throughout the country, with certain core competencies."[37]

Gradually the COVID-19 mortality rate began to fall. In a later study, from March to August 2020, of 1,000 hospitals across the United States, 15% of hospitalized patients died, and of those discharged, 60% went home, 15% to a long-term care facility (LTCF), 10% to home health, and 4% to hospice (see Table 1.1).[38] Readmission correlated with age >65 years, multiple comorbidities, and discharge to a skilled nursing facility or home care.

In a 60-day, follow-up study of 1,650 patients admitted to 38 hospitals in Michigan, 24% died and 15% of hospital survivors had been readmitted.[39] More than one-half reported that they were mildly or moderately affected emotionally by the illness. In a Veterans Administration (VA) study of 2,200 patients hospitalized with COVID from March 1 to June 1, 2020, 31% were

[36] Gupta S, Hayek SS, Wang W, Chan L, Mathews KS, Melamed ML, et al. Factors associated with death in critically ill patients with coronavirus disease 2019 in the US. *JAMA Intern Med.* 2020;180(11):1436–1446. doi:10.1001/jamainternmed.2020.3596.

[37] Lamas DJ. "If I hadn't been transferred, I would have died." *The New York Times.* August 4, 2020.

[38] Lavery AM, Preston LE, Ko JY, Chevinsky JR, DeSisto CL, Pennington AF, et al. Characteristics of hospitalized COVID-19 patients discharged and experiencing same-hospital readmission—United States, March–August 2020. *MMWR.* 2020;69:1695–1699.

[39] Chopra V, Flanders SA, O'Malley M, Malani AN, Prescott HC. Sixty-day outcomes among patients hospitalized with COVID-19. *Ann Intern Med.* November 11, 2020. doi.org/10.7326/M20-5661.

Table 1.1 Characteristics of Patients Discharged after Severe COVID-19 Infection

Characteristic	Sent Home	To LTCF	Home Health	Hospice
% discharged	60	15	10	4
Length of index hospital stay (median days)	4	8	8	7
Median age, yrs	53	76	68	83
ICU admission, %	35	42	45	53
% readmitted	7	15	12	4

Modified from Lavery AM, Preston LE, Ko JY, Chevinsky JR, DeSisto CL, Pennington AF, et al. Characteristics of hospitalized COVID-19 patients discharged and experiencing same-hospital readmission. United States, March–August 2020. *MMWR*. 2020;69:1695–1699.

treated in the ICU and 18% died.[40] Twenty percent of the discharged patients were readmitted within 60 days and 10% died.

The hospital mortality rate from COVID-19 decreased further during the summer of 2020. Mortality in 4,700 hospitalized patients in New York City dropped from 33% in April to 2% in the late June 2020 (Figure 1.2).[41] In the United Kingdom the 30-day mortality of 30%–40% for people admitted to critical care in April 2020 dropped to 10%–25% for those admitted in May 2020.[42] Dr. John Dennis, a lead investigator of that UK study, noted, "In late March, four in 10 people in intensive care were dying. By the end of June, survival was over 80 percent. It was really quite dramatic."[43]

The decreased mortality was, in part, related to a decrease in the age of hospitalized patients. The median age of all confirmed COVID infections in the United States was 46 years on May 1, 2020, compared to 38 years at the

[40] Donnelly JP, Wang XQ, Iwashyna TJ, Prescott HC. Readmission and death after initial hospital discharge among patients with COVID-19 in a large multihospital system. *JAMA Network*. 2021;325(3):304–306. doi: 10.1001/jama.2020.21465.

[41] Horwitz LI, Jones SA, Cerfolio RJ, Francois F, Greco J, Rudy B, et al. Trends in COVID-19 risk-adjusted mortality rates. *J Hosp Med*. October 23, 2020. doi: 10.12788/jhm.3552.

[42] Dennis J, McGovern A, Vollmer S, Mateen BA. Improving COVID-19 critical care mortality over time in England: A national study, March to June 2020. *medRxiv*. Accessed March 12, 2021. https://doi.org/10.1101/2020.07.30.20165134.

[43] Rabin RC. Death rates have dropped for seriously ill Covid patients. *The New York Times*. October 29, 2020.

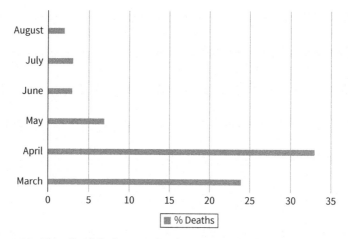

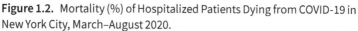

Figure 1.2. Mortality (%) of Hospitalized Patients Dying from COVID-19 in New York City, March–August 2020.

From: Horwitz LI, Jones SA, Cerfolio RJ, Francois F, Greco J, Rudy B, et al. Trends in COVID-19 risk- adjusted mortality rates. *J Hosp Med.* October 23, 2020.

end of August.[44] The median age for the hospitalized patients decreased from 67 years in March 2020 to 49 years in June. In Houston, Texas, patients hospitalized between May 16 to July 7, 2020, compared to those hospitalized between March 13 and May 15, 2020, were younger, had a lower burden of comorbidities, and a decrease in the case fatality rate (CFR).[45]

The decrease in CFR was also, in part, related to improved care, including treatment for COVID-related hypercoagulability. Thrombotic events were found in more than one-third of COVID-hospitalized patients.[46] Deep venous thrombosis (DVT) typically occurred 4–10 days after hospitalization, and one-third of DVTs were associated with pulmonary embolism.[47]

[44] Boehmer TK, DeVies J, Caruso E, van Santen KL, Tang S, Black C, et al. Changing age distribution of the COVID-19 pandemic—United States, May–August 2020. *MMWR.* 2020;69:1404–1409. http://dx.doi.org/0.15585/mmwr.mm6939e1.

[45] Vahidy FS, Drews AL, Masud FN, Schwartz RL, Askary B, Boom ML, et al. Characteristics and outcomes of COVID-19 patients during initial peak and resurgence in the Houston metropolitan area. *JAMA.* 2020;324:998–1000. doi:10.1001/jama.2020.15301.

[46] Piazza G, Morrow DA. Diagnosis, management, and pathophysiology of arterial and venous thrombosis in COVID-19. *JAMA.* November 23, 2020.

[47] Gomez-Mesa JE, Galindo S, Montes MC, Munoz Martin AJ. Thrombosis and coagulopathy in COVID-19. *Curr Probs Cardiol.* 2021 Mar;46(3):100742. doi: 10.1016/j.cpcardiol.2020.100742.

DVTs and pulmonary embolism rates ranged from 14% to 30% in COVID patients with severe or critical disease but were lower in later series when anticoagulation was begun immediately in all patients hospitalized with COVID-19.[48] Pulmonary embolisms associated with COVID infection typically form in the more peripheral pulmonary arteries. Histologic analysis of pulmonary vessels in patients with COVID-19 reveals widespread thrombosis and a diffuse microangiopathy.[49] Alveolar capillary microthrombi were nine times as prevalent in patients with COVID-19 as in patients with influenza and the amount of new blood vessel growth was three times as high as that in the lungs from patients with influenza.

Thromboprophylaxis, typically with low-molecular weight heparins or fondaparinux, became the standard of care in every hospitalized patient. Full-dose anticoagulation is essential in patients needing respiratory support with extracorporeal membrane oxygenation (ECMO) in order to prevent clotting of vascular access. Because there has been a high rate of thrombotic events despite thromboprophylaxis in critically ill patients, some experts have recommended high doses of anticoagulants and extending anticoagulation after hospital discharge. More studies are being done to determine optimal antithrombotic therapy in hospitalized patients, at discharge, and in nonhospitalized patients at high risk for thrombosis.

Results from the UK-based RECOVERY trial in June 2020 demonstrated that treatment with corticosteroids reduced fatality by one-third in patients receiving mechanical ventilation and by one-fifth in patients getting supplemental oxygen.[50] Corticosteroids soon were administered to all critically ill COVID patients around the world. Remdesivir shortened the time to recovery in adults hospitalized with COVID-19.[51] The use of interleukin-6

[48] McBane RD, Torres Roldan VD, Niven AS, Pruthi RK, Moreno Franco P, Linderbaum JA, et al. Anticoagulation in COVID-19: A systematic review, meta-analysis, and rapid guidance from the Mayo Clinic. *Mayo Clin Proc.* 2020 Nov;95:2467–2486. doi: 10.1016/j.mayocp.2020.08.030.

[49] Ackermann M, Verleden SE, Kuehnel M, Haverich A, Welte T, Laenger F, et al. Pulmonary vascular endothelialitis, thrombosis, and angiogenesis on Covid-19. *N Engl J Med.* 2020 Jul 9;383:120–128. doi: 10.1056/NEJMoa2015432.

[50] RECOVERY Collaborative Group. Dexamethasone in hospitalized patients with Covid-19: Preliminary report. *N Engl J Med.* 2020 Jul 17;384:693–704. doi:10.1056/NEJMoa2021436.

[51] Beigel JH, Tomashek KM, Dodd LE, Mehta AK, Zingman BS, Kalil AC, et al. Remdesivir for the treatment of Covid-19-Final report. *N Engl J Med.* 2020;383:1813–1826. doi: 10.1056/NEJMoa2007764.

receptor antagonists in critically ill hospitalized patients decreased hospital mortality.[52]

Increased expertise in ICU management, such as awake proning, was also an important factor in improved patient outcome. Dr. Leora Horwitz discussed the decreased CFR in New York: "We don't have a magic bullet cure, but we have a lot, a lot of little things, that add up. We understand better when people need to be on ventilators and when they don't, and what complications to watch for, like blood clots and kidney failure. We understand how to watch for oxygen levels even before patients are in the hospital, so we can bring them in earlier. And of course, we understand that steroids are helpful, and possibly some other medications. This is still a high death rate, much higher than we see for flu or other respiratory diseases. I don't want to pretend this is benign. But it definitely is something that has given me hope."[53]

Possibly the most important factor in the decreased hospital mortality rate from COVID-19 was the gradual decline in community infection rate in the first 6 months of the pandemic. When hospitals and ICUs were overwhelmed with patients, their care suffered. When there were plenty of beds, ventilators, oxygen, nurses, and doctors, their care improved. In a study of 40,000 adults admitted to 955 hospitals throughout the United States, 94% of the hospitals had a significant decreased CFR during those initial 6 months.[54] The mean overall mortality rate decreased by 50%, and this correlated with declines in county-level case rates. Dr. Tom Inglesby, the director of the Center for Health Security at Johns Hopkins University, warned, "If you compare the number of people who are dying from every 100 cases diagnosed in the U.S., it's obviously substantially lower than it was in the summertime, and a lot lower than it was in the springtime. If hospitals that aren't prepared for large numbers of people have to deal with a large influx of Covid patients, or small

[52] Gordon AC, Mouncey PR, Al-Beidh F, Rowan KM, Nicol AD, Arabi YM, et al. Interleukin-6 receptor antagonists in critically ill patients with Covid-19-Preliminary report. *medRxiv*. January 7, 2021. doi: https://doi.org/10.1101/2021.01.07.21249390.

[53] Rabin RC. Death rates have dropped for seriously ill Covid patients. *The New York Times*. October 29, 2020.

[54] Asch DA, Sheils NE, Islam MN, Chen Y, Werner RM, Buresh J, et al. Variation in hospital mortality rates for patients admitted with COVID-19 during the first 6 months of the pandemic. *JAMA Intern Med*. December 22, 2020. 2021;181(4):471–478. doi: 10.1001/jamainternmed.2020.8193.

hospitals get pulled into it, we should expect that mortality could change unfortunately. That's a warning."[55]

And, of course, these dire predictions proved correct. The fall/winter 2020 surge involved every county and state in the United States. The virus invaded cities not previously hit hard and circled back to those that had contained the pandemic in March through May. Dr. Lamas captured the increased dread that hospital-based physicians felt in the fall with this new COVID surge, "But now, as the air grows crisp here in Boston and the nation endures an average of 59,000 new cases a day—levels that we have not seen since August—the threat of a 'third wave,' or a winter surge, of this virus builds. And we find ourselves once again in limbo, haunted by the ghosts of the spring while steeling ourselves for the resurgence of illness and isolation that might come. So we control what we can. Looking ahead to the possibility of another surge here in the Northeast, as the cold air drives us indoors, we refine our protocols and procedures. We arrange schedules. We make cautious plans to see the people we love. We laugh when we can, even if nothing is actually funny, because that is better than the alternative."[56]

Throughout the United States, 2021 was ushered in with an alarming increase in COVID-19 cases, hospitalizations, and deaths. Once again, the system was overwhelmed. The 7-day average for daily deaths tripled with more than 4,000 deaths from COVID in the United States on January 7, 2021.[57] As 2020 ended, more than 340,000 Americans had died and COVID-19 became the leading cause of death in the United States, surpassing heart disease and cancer.

On January 4, 2021, the United Kingdom issued strict new national lockdown orders, as 60,000 cases per day were recorded and 26,000 COVID-19 patients were in hospitals, an increase of 30% from the prior week. More than 75,000 had died from COVID-19 in the United Kingdom. That same day, 128,000 patients were hospitalized in Los Angeles County, and ambulances were being turned away from hospitals that were running out of oxygen supplies. Dr. Robert Kim-Farley, a medical epidemiologist at the UCLA Fielding School of Public Health, said, "When you get to that level of volume being

---

[55] Rabin RC. Death rates have dropped for seriously ill Covid patients. *The New York Times.* October 29, 2020.

[56] Lamas DJ. Doctors are dreading the winter. *The New York Times.* October 27, 2020.

[57] Koh HK, Geller AC, VanderWeele TJ. Deaths from COVID-19. *JAMA.* December 17, 2020. 2020;325(2):133–134. doi: 10.1001/jama.2020.25381.

pumped through, some of the pipes start to freeze up. You start running out of oxygen tanks that patients need to be sent home and discharged. As the cases keep increasing, you're going to see those kinds of effects start to pile up. ICU beds get full. The ER gets backed up. Ambulances have nowhere to take patients. You get severe, chronic staffing shortages. Elective surgeries get canceled again. The ability to care simply degrades. We're no longer a wave or surge or surge upon a surge. We're really in the middle of a viral tsunami."[58]

These surges in infections and hospitalizations finally subsided as COVID-19 vaccination rates in the United States picked up in March–June 2021.

Impact on Non-COVID-19 Patients with Urgent Medical Conditions

The pandemic also had an adverse effect on urgent non-COVID diseases. During 2020, there were 370,000 increased deaths in the United States compared to the previous few years.[59] More than a quarter of these excess deaths were from diseases not directly linked to COVID-19. There were 15% more deaths attributed to diabetes, 12% from Alzheimer's disease and dementia, 11% attributed to hypertension, 11% pneumonia, 6% coronary heart disease, and 5% stroke. Many of these excess deaths were an indirect result of the pandemic.

Forty percent of US adults had avoided medical care because of concerns about COVID during the pandemic.[60] This included 12% who avoided urgent or emergency care and 32% avoiding routine care. Urgent care was avoided more in people with more than two underlying medical conditions, in Black and Hispanic people, and in those with disabilities. One US survey found a 34% decrease in hospital admissions for common cardiac, gastrointestinal, neurologic, and urologic disorders during April and May 2020 compared to the same time frame in the prior year.[61] In New York City, it was

[58] Nirappil F, Wan W. Los Angeles is running out of oxygen for patients as Covid hospitalizations hit record high nationwide. *The Washington Post.* January 5, 2021.

[59] Lu D. 2020 was especially deadly: Covid wasn't the only culprit. *The New York Times.* December 13, 2020.

[60] Wong LE, Hawkins JE, Langness S, Murrell KL, Iris P, Sammann A. Where are all the patients? *NEJM Catalyst.* May 14, 2020. doi: 10.1056/CAT.20.0193.

[61] Blecker S, Jones SA, Petrilli CM, Admon AJ, Weerahandi H, Francois F, Horwitz LI. Hospitalizations for chronic diseases and acute conditions in the time of COVID-19. *JAMA Int Med.* October 26, 2020. 2021;181(2):269–271. doi: 10.1001/jamainternmed.2020.3978.

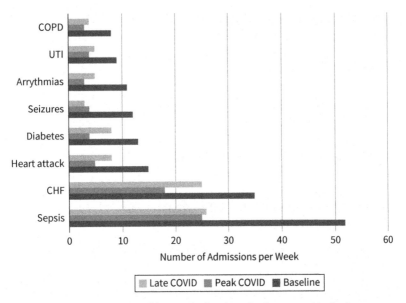

Figure 1.3. Decrease in Weekly Hospitalizations for Common Medical Disorders during Peak and Late COVID-19 Pandemic.

From: Blecker S, Jones SA, Petrilli CM, Admon AJ, Weerahandi H, Francois F, et al. Hospitalizations for chronic disease and acute conditions in the time of COVID-19. *JAMA Intern Med*. October 26, 2020.

estimated that more than one-quarter of the 24,000 excess deaths from mid-March to May were "from delays in seeking or obtaining lifesaving care."[62] Weekly hospitalization rates for the most common diseases, including sepsis, congestive heart failure (CHF), heart attacks, cardiac arrhythmias, complications of diabetes, seizures, urinary tract infections (UTIs), and chronic obstructive pulmonary disease (COPD), decreased significantly during the peak COVID pandemic and that trend persisted even late in the pandemic (Figure 1.3).[63]

[62] Fink S. Hospitals move into next phase as New York passes viral peak. *The New York Times*. May 20, 2020.

[63] Blecker S, Jones SA, Petrilli CM, Admon AJ, Weerahandi H, Francois F, et al. Hospitalizations for chronic disease and acute conditions in the time of COVID-19. *JAMA Intern Med*. October 26, 2020. 2021;181(2):269–271.

Dr. Thomas Lee, Editor-in-Chief of *NEJM Catalyst Innovations in Care*, said in April 2020, "Like everyone else in health care, I think about Covid-19 all day long. I'm exhausted from reading emails about Covid, but I don't feel like reading anything else. I spend my day on calls and emails about Covid patients, and don't have much bandwidth left for patients without Covid-19. But, of course, they are out there. They feel like they are invisible—they actually apologize for disturbing us at this terrible time. And even though they don't have the virus, they are being deeply affected by the Covid-19 pandemic. From my own panel of patients and those of my friends, I could tell you about the patient with debilitating back pain for whom surgery has been put off until . . . who knows when? Or multiple patients with problems for whom emergency department or urgent care visits would ordinarily be recommended, but who are now deciding to hope for the best at home. Their suffering is real, as is that of their families. They don't have to be casualties of war."[64]

During the first 3 months of the pandemic in the United States, emergency department visits were down 42%.[65] There were 23% fewer ER visits for heart attacks, 20% for strokes, and 10% for blood sugar crisis. Dr. Harlan Krumholz, a cardiologist at Yale New Haven Hospital, asked, "Where are all the patients with heart attacks and stroke? They are missing from our hospitals . . . cardiologists are seeing a 40 percent to 60 percent reduction in admissions for heart attacks; about 20 percent reported more than a 60 percent reduction. Time to treatment dictates the outcomes for people with heart attacks and strokes. These deaths may not be labeled Covid-19 deaths, but surely, they are collateral damage."[66] Out-of-hospital cardiac arrests (OHCAs) doubled during the pandemic compared to the previous year (Figure 1.4).[67] The proportion of OHCA calls for patients who died in the field increased by 40% during the pandemic. A greater number of these

[64] Lee TH. The invisible patient: Caring for those without Covid-19. *N Engl J Med*. April 27, 2020. https://catalyst.nejm.org/doi/full/10.1056/CAT.20.0139

[65] Lange SJ, Ritchey MD, Goodman AB, Dias T, Twentyman E, Fuld J, et al. Potential indirect effects of the COVID-19 pandemic on use of emergency departments for acute life-threatening conditions—United States, January–May 2020. *MMWR*. June 26, 2020. 2020:69;795–800.

[66] Krumholz HM. Where have all the heart attacks gone? *The New York Times*. April 6, 2020.

[67] Nickles AV, Oostema A, Allen J, O'Brien SL, Demel SL, Reeves MJ. Comparison of out-of-hospital cardiac arrests and fatalities in the Metro Detroit area during the COVID-19 pandemic with previous-year-events. *JAMA Netw Open*. 2021;4(1):e2032331. doi: 10.1001/jamanetworkopen.2020.32331.

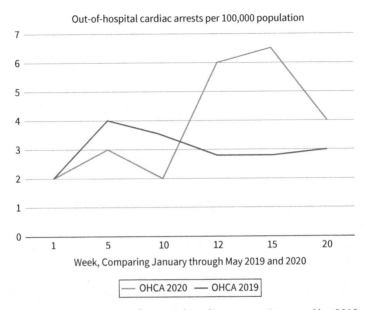

Figure 1.4. Comparing Out-of-Hospital Cardiac Arrests, January–May 2019 vs. 2020, Metro Detroit.

From: Nickles AV, Oostema A, Allen J, O'Brien SL, Demel SL, Reeves MJ. Comparison of out-of-hospital cardiac arrests and fatalities in the Metro Detroit area during the COVID-19 pandemic with previous-year-events. *JAMA Netw Open*. 2021;4(1):e2032331. doi:10.1001/jamanetworkopen.2020.32331.

OHCAs occurred in older individuals and those in long-term care facilities in 2020 compared to 2019.

In every part of the United States, the number of patients who underwent magnetic resonance imaging (MRI) and ultrasound for possible stroke decreased by 40% during the early months of the pandemic.[68] A California community hospital reported that since the pandemic began their stroke patients have all arrived too late to receive tissue plasminogen activator (TPA).[69] These patients were worried that "hospitals are crawling with

[68] Wong LE, Hawkins JE, Langress S, Murrell KL, Iris P, Sammann A. Where are all the patients? Addressing Covid-19 fear to encourage sick patients to seek emergency care. *N Engl J Med*. May 14, 2020.

[69] Wong LE, Hawkins JE, Langress S, Murrell KL, Iris P, Sammann A. Where are all the patients? Addressing Covid-19 fear to encourage sick patients to seek emergency care. *N Engl J Med*. May 14, 2020.

Covid-19". There was a 40% decrease in stroke admissions to a comprehensive stroke center in the United Kingdom during March 15, 2020, to April 14, 2020, compared to the previous year.[70]

Most clinicians thought that the downtick in hospital care for emergency medical conditions reflected the public's initial fear of catching COVID-19 and anticipated that this would subside over time. However, restoring public confidence has been slow. As noted by Dr. Pauline Chen, "For much of the spring and summer, the halls and parking lots were eerily empty. I wondered if people were staying home and getting sicker, and I imagined that in a few months' time these patients, once they became too ill to manage on their own, might flood the emergency rooms, wards and I.C.U.s, in a non-Covid wave. But more than seven months into the pandemic, there are still no lines of patients in the halls. While my colleagues and I are busier than we were in March, there has been no pent-up overflow of people with crushing chest pain, debilitating shortness of breath or fevers and wet, rattling coughs."[71] Even when office visits and elective surgery opened up in July–September 2020, hospital admissions were still 20% lower than the previous year.[72] Non-COVID admissions were significantly lower for pneumonia, asthma/COPD, sepsis, and acute ST-elevation myocardial infarction. The study's lead author, Dr. John Birkmeyer, commented, "We found it staggering that such a high number of patients who might have been hospitalized for serious issues just kind of disappeared. You have to wonder, where did they all go?"[73]

The director of the National Cancer Institute forecast that reduced screenings and diagnostic delays will result in 10,000 excess deaths from breast and colorectal cancer in the United States during the next 10 years.[74] In the United Kingdom, comparing July 2019 to July 2020, there was an eighty-fold increase in patients waiting more than a year for treatment and a fourfold drop in cancer patients receiving their first treatment within

[70] Padmanabhan N, Natarajan I, Gunston R, Raseta M, Roffe C. Impact of COVID-19 on stroke admissions, treatments, and outcomes at a comprehensive stroke centre in the United Kingdom. *Neurol Sci.* 2020 Oct 6;1–6. doi: 10.1007/s10072-020-04775-x.

[71] Chen PW. Where have all the patients gone? *The New York Times.* October 20, 2020.

[72] Birkmeyer JD, Barnato A, Birkmeyer N, Bessler R, Skinner J. The impact of the COVID-19 pandemic on hospital admissions in the United States. *Health Affairs.* September 24, 2020. 2020;39.11.

[73] Birkmeyer JD, Barnato A, Birkmeyer N, Bessler R, Skinner J. The impact of the COVID-19 pandemic on hospital admissions in the United States. *Health Affairs.* September 24, 2020. 2020;39.11.

[74] Sharpless NE. COVID-19 and cancer. *Science.* 2020;368:1290.

2 months after first referral.[75] During the early months of the pandemic, urgent referrals for cancer care declined by 70% and chemotherapy by 40% in the United Kingdom, and these numbers were still down at 45% and 31% on May 31, 2020.[76] Using real-time data and disease modeling, these investigators estimated that there will be between 7,000 and 18,000 excess deaths in UK cancer patients over the next year. Dr. Nahid Bhadelie, medical director of Boston University School of Medicine Special Pathogens Unit, cautioned, "This data underlines the importance of not letting our health systems get to the point where they are so overwhelmed that it spills over and affects people with other medical conditions in our community."[77] Only time will tell what the long-term outcome will be for the millions of people who missed their regular healthcare during the pandemic.

[75] Griffin S. Covid-19: Waiting times in England reach record highs. *BMJ.* 2020;370:m3557.
[76] Lai AG, Pasea L, Banerjee A, Hall G, Denaxas S, Chang WH, et al. Estimated impact of the COVID-19 pandemic on cancer services and excess 1-year mortality in people with cancer and multimorbidity: Near real time data on cancer care, cancer deaths and a population-based cohort study. *BMJ Open.* November 17, 2020. 2020;10:e043828. doi: 10.1136/bmjopen-2020-043828.
[77] Thebault R, Bernstein L, Ba Tran A, Shin Y. Heart conditions drove spike in deaths beyond those attributed to covid-19, analysis shows. *The Washington Post.* July 2, 2020.

2
Risk Factors

Age

The two most important risk factors for COVID-19 disease severity and death are age and comorbidities. These are interwoven since the prevalence of every chronic illness increases with aging. More than 75% of older Americans have at least two chronic medical conditions—primarily heart disease, stroke, diabetes, and cancer—which account for two-thirds of our yearly mortality.[1]

In the United States there has been a striking correlation between COVID-19 mortality and age, with three-quarters of deaths occurring in those 65 years and older (Figure 2.1).[2] The fatality rate in older patients was especially alarming early in the pandemic. In the first 72,000 cases from China, the overall case fatality rate (CFR) was 2.3%, but it was 8% in those aged 70–79 years and 15% in those >79 years.[3] In Italy, the oldest country in Europe, the CFR in March and April 2020 was 7.2, and 51% of COVID infections were in people >60 years, including 19% in those >80 years.[4] In the United States from February to March 16, 45% of COVID hospitalizations, 53% of ICU admissions, and 80% of deaths were among adults aged ≥65 years with the highest fatalities among persons aged ≥85 years.[5] Adults over age 65 years had a twenty-three-fold greater risk of dying from COVID compared to those <65.[6] In a UK study of more than 20,000 COVID-hospitalized

[1] National Council on Aging. "Healthy Aging Facts. 2020."

[2] CDC COVID Data Tracker. COVID.CDC.gov. December 31, 2020.

[3] Wu Z, McGoogan JM. Characteristics of and important lessons from the coronavirus disease 2019 (COVID-19) outbreak in China. *JAMA*. 2020;323:1239–1242.

[4] Volpato S, Landi F, Antonelli Incalzi RA. A frail health care system for an old population: Lesson from the COVID-19 outbreak in Italy. *J Gerontol*. September 16 2020; 75(9):e126–e127.

[5] CDC. Severe outcomes among patients with coronavirus disease 2019 (COVID-19), United States, February 12–March 16, 2020. *MMWR*. March 27, 2020;69(12):343–346.

[6] Mueller AL, McNamara MS, Sinclair DA. Why does COVID-19 disproportionately affect older people? *Aging*. May 29, 2020;12(10):9959–9981.

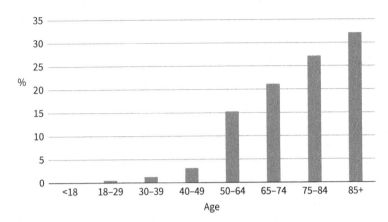

Figure 2.1. Percentage of Deaths by Age Category in the United States.
From: CDC COVID Data Tracker. COVID.CDC.gov. December 31, 2020.

patients, age was the most important mortality risk factor.[7] The mean mortality hazard ratio increased with each 10 years of age, from 2.6 at age 50–59, 5 at age 60–69, 8.5 at age 70–79, and to 11 at age >80 years (Figure 2.2). The UK OpenSAFELY study tracked the risk factors associated with 11,000 COVID-19 related deaths in a registry of 17 million adult patients.[8] This very large study reaffirmed the prior studies demonstrating that age is the most prominent COVID risk factor. People over the age of 80 had a twenty-fold increased mortality risk compared to 50–59-year-olds.

Aging is associated with a reduction in natural killer cell activity and a blunted macrophage response.[9] As we age, there are decreased naïve T cells and a reduced ability to convert those T cells to memory cells.[10] This immunosenescence triggers a hyperactivation of inflammatory cells.[11] Such

[7] Docherty AB, Harrison EM, Green CA, Hardwick H, Pius R, Norman L, et al. Features of 20,133 UK patients in hospital with Covid-19 using the ISARIC WHO Clinical Characterization Protocol: Prospective observational study. *BMJ*. May 22, 2020. 2020;369:m1985.

[8] Williamson EJ, Walker AJ, Goldacre B, Bhaskaran K, Bacon S, Bates C, et al. Factors associated with COVID-19-related death using OpenSafely. *Nature*. 2020;584:430–436.

[9] Mueller AL, McNamara MS, Sinclar DA. Why does COVID-19 disproportionately affect older people? *Aging*. May 29, 20202020;369:m1985.

[10] Salimi S, Hamlyn JM. COVID-19 and crosstalk with the hallmarks of aging. *J Gerontol A Biol Sci Med Sci*. September 16 2020;75(9):e34–e41. doi: 10.1093/gerona/glaa149.

[11] Mahbub S, Brubaker AL, Kovacs EJ. Aging of the innate immune system: An update. *Curr Immunol Rev*. 2011;7:104–115.

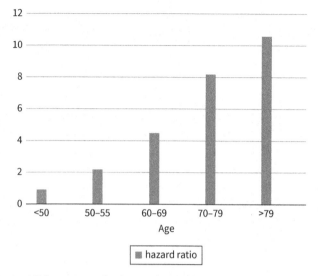

Figure 2.2. COVID-19 Mortality (Hazard Ratio) by Age, United Kingdom. From: Docherty AB, Harrison EM, Green CA, et al. Features of 20,133 UK patients in hospital with covid-19 using the ISARIC WHO Clinical Characterization Protocol: Prospective observational study. *BMJ.* May 22, 2020.

age-related hyperactivity, termed "inflammaging," has been implicated in the "cytokine storm" characteristic of severe COVID infections.[12]

Children rarely develop moderate or severe symptoms and as of December 21, 2020, with 225,000 deaths in adults, there had been only 187 deaths from COVID-19 in children in the United States, including only 57 in children under the age of 5 years.[13] In a series of 1,165 infants tested for SARS-CoV-2 infection at a medical center in Canada, 2% were positive.[14] One-third required hospitalization, but the illness was mild with a predominance of gastrointestinal symptoms. As in adults, children with severe symptoms have usually had underlying chronic medical conditions, such as diabetes,

[12] Mahbub S, Brubaker AL, Kovacs EJ. Aging of the innate immune system: An update. *Curr Immunol Rev.* 2011;7:104–115.

[13] American Academy of Pediatrics. Children and COVID-19: State data report: 9/10/20.

[14] Panetta L, Proulx C, Drouin O, Autmizguine J, Luu TM, Quach C, et al. Clinical characteristics and disease severity among infants with SARS-CoV-2 infection in Montreal, Quebec, Canada. *JAMA Netw Open.* 2020;3(12):e2030470. December 14, 2020. doi: 10.1001/jamanetworkopen.2020.30470.

cardiovascular disease, developmental conditions, and asthma. Dr. Larry Steinman, a professor of pediatrics and neurology at Stanford University School of Medicine, noted, "It seems notable that this pandemic, which has had so much of a toll in mortality and morbidity, does seem to spare kids in a dramatic way."[15] ACE2 receptors increase in the lungs with age, and young children have fewer ACE2 receptors than adults.[16]

Multisystem inflammatory disease in children (MIS-C) had been reported in 1,097 cases in the United States as of October 15, 2020.[17] There had been 20 deaths. The average age was 8 years and more than 75% were in Hispanic, Latino, or Black children. MIS-C typically presented 2–4 weeks after COVID infection. MIS-C is considered to be an immune-mediated systemic disease. Patients have fever and multisystem disease, which may include cardiac, renal, dermatologic, gastrointestinal, and neurologic involvement. Laboratory tests include an elevated C-reactive protein (CRP), erythrocyte sedimentation rate (ESR), fibrinogen, procalcitonin, d-dimer, ferritin, lactic acid dehydrogenase (LDH) or interleukin 6 (IL-6), elevated neutrophils, reduced lymphocytes, and low albumin. Despite the severity of symptoms, the majority of children recover fully, usually responding well to anti-inflammatory/immunosuppressive medications.

In a series of 186 patients with MIS-C from 26 states in the United States, 73% had been previously healthy and 88% were hospitalized.[18] Median age was 8 years, and 62% were males. Organ system involvement included gastrointestinal in 92%, cardiovascular in 80%, hematologic in 76%, mucocutaneous in 74%, and respiratory in 70%. Eighty percent required ICU care, and 20% required mechanical ventilation. Kawasaki's disease–like features were present in 40%. The average duration of hospitalization was 7 days, and four patients (2%) died. MIS was reported in 27 adults, age

[15] Bernstein L. Child deaths from covid-19 remain remarkably low eight months into U.S. pandemic. *The Washington Post.* September 25, 2020.

[16] Santesmasses D, Castro JP, Zenin AA, Shindyapina AV, Gerashchenko MV, Zhang B, et al. COVID-19 is an emergent disease of aging. *Aging Cell.* October 19, 2020. 2020;(10):e13230. doi: 10.1111/acel.13230.

[17] CDC. Health department-reported cases of multisystem inflammatory syndrome in children (MIS-C) in the United States. October 15, 2020.

[18] Feldstein LR, Rose EB, Horwitz SM, Collins JP, Newhams MM, Son MB. Multisystem inflammatory syndrome in U.S. children and adolescents. *N Engl J Med.* June 29, 2020. 2020;383:334–346. doi: 10.1056/NEJMoa2021680.

21–50 years.[19] The case definition required severe extrapulmonary organ system involvement with absence of significant pulmonary disease. All had cardiac disease, and most had gastrointestinal involvement. Ten required ICU care, and two died.

Adolescents and young adults also have had predominately mild COVID-19 infections. In a series of 736 US sailors, median age 25 years, diagnosed with COVID-19, cough was present in 45%, cold-like symptoms in 53%, anosmia in 37%, headache in 34%, but fever in just 8% and dyspnea in only 3%.[20] A total of 6 of the 736 patients were hospitalized, and there was one death. In a prospective study of nonhospitalized household contacts with a COVID-19-infected person, fever was present in only 19%, and 17% were initially asymptomatic, although all eventually developed symptoms.[21] Respiratory symptoms were less common in children and young adults.

The CFR in young adults, under age 40, ranges from 1% to 3%. This may be underestimated since there were 12,000 more deaths in the 18–44 age group in the United States from March through the end of July 2020 than during prior years.[22] This age group still accounts for only 3% of US COVID deaths, but the authors of that study warned, "But what we believed before about the relative harmlessness of Covid-19 among younger adults has simply not been borne out by emerging data. We need to amend our messaging and our policies now. Outreach in the coming weeks and months is imperative. We need to tell young people that they are at risk and that they need to wear masks and make safer choices about social distancing."[23]

[19] Morris S, Schwartz N, Patel P, Abbo L, Beauchamps L, Balan S, et al. Case series of multisystem inflammatory syndrome in adults associated with SARS-CoV-2 Infection-United Kingdom and United States, March–August 2020. 2020;69(40):1450–1456 *MMWR*. October 9, 2020.

[20] Alvarado GR, Pierson BC, Teemer ES, Gama HC, Cole RD, Jang SS. Symptom characterization and outcome of sailors in isolation after a COVID-19 outbreak on a US aircraft carrier. *JAMA*. 2020;3:e2020981. doi:10.1001/jamanetworkopen.2020.20981.

[21] Yousaf AR, Duca LM, Chu V, Reses HE, Fajans M, Rabold EM, et al. A prospective cohort study in non-hospitalized household contacts with SARS-CoV-2 infection: Symptom profiles and symptom change over time. *Clin Infect Dis*. July 28, 2020. doi:10.1093/cid/ciaa1072.

[22] Faust JS, Krumholz HM, Du C, Mayes KD, Lin A, Gilman C, et al. All-cause excess mortality and COVID-19 related mortality among US adults aged 25–44 years, March–July 2020. *JAMA*. December 16, 2020. 2021;325(8):785–787.

[23] Faust J, Krumholz HM, Walensky RP. Yes, young people are dying of Covid. *The New York Times*. December 16, 2020.

Comorbidities, Including Obesity and Diabetes

It is difficult to tease out the effect of age itself from that of age-related comorbidity. The UK OpenSAFELY study found an increased mortality risk with obesity, diabetes, severe asthma, chronic pulmonary and cardiac disease, cancer, liver disease, stroke, dementia, renal dysfunction, and autoimmune diseases.[24] In a study from the United States, comorbidities were present in 27% of COVID patients not requiring hospitalization compared to 71% of those requiring hospitalization and 78% of ICU patients.[25] Almost 90% of 5,700 Covid-19 patients admitted between March 1 and April 4, 2020, to a dozen hospitals in New York City, Long Island, and Westchester County, had two or more chronic medical conditions.[26] In more than 20,000 UK hospitalized COVID patients, 78% had at least one comorbidity, including 31% with cardiac disease, 21% with diabetes, 18% with chronic pulmonary disease, and 16% with chronic kidney disease.[27] A US study of 31,461 COVID-infected patients reported that cardiovascular disease, chronic pulmonary disease, dementia, renal disease, metastatic cancer, and chronic liver disease had the highest adjusted odds ratio of death from COVID-19.[28]

The odds ratio for severe and fatal COVID-19 in a population study in Scotland were 5.4 for neurological disease, 4.1 for chronic kidney disease, 3.6 for chronic liver disease, 2.75 for type 2 diabetes, 2.0 for lower respiratory disease, 1.5 for ischemic heart disease, and 2.2 for other cardiac disease.[29] Seventy-eight percent of severe cases had at least one chronic medical condition and that included 51% of patients <40 years.

---

[24] Williamson EJ, Walker AJ, Goldacre B, Bhaskaran K, Bacon S, Bates C, et al. Factors associated with COVID-19-related death using OpenSafely. *Nature.* 2020;584:430–436.

[25] Chow N, Fleming-Dutra K, Gierke R, Hall A, Hughes M, Pilishvili T, et al. Preliminary estimates of the prevalence of selected underlying health conditions among patients with coronavirus disease 2019—United States, February 12–March 28, 2020. *MMWR.* 2020;3;69:382.

[26] Rabin RC. Nearly all patients hospitalized with Covid-19 had chronic health issues, Study Finds. *The New York Times.* April 23, 2020.

[27] Docherty AB, Harrison EM, Green CA, Hardwick H, Pius R, Norman L, et al. Features of 20,133 UK patients in hospital with covid-19 using the ISARIC WHO Clinical Characterization Protocol: Prospective observational study. *BMJ.* May 22, 2020. 2020;369:m1985.

[28] Harrison SL, Fazio-Eynulayeva E, Lane DA, Underhill P, Lip GYH. Comorbidities associated with mortality in 31,461 adults with COVID-19 in the United States: A federated electronic medical record analysis. *PLoS Med.* 2020;17:e1003321. doi: 10.1371/journal.pmed.1003321.

[29] McKeigue PM, Weir A, Bishop J, McGurnaghan SJ, Kennedy S, McAllister D, et al. Rapid epidemiological analysis of comorbidities and treatments as risk factors for COVID-19 in Scotland (REACT-SCOT): A population-based case-control study. *PLoS Med.* October 20, 2020. 2020;17(10):e1003374. doi: 10.1371/journal.pmed.1003374.

Obesity has been an important risk factor for COVID-19 infection as well as for COVID-related morbidity and mortality. This has been true in most countries, although not in those countries with a lower population prevalence of obesity, such as China.[30] The United States has the highest rates of obesity in the industrialized world, with more than 40% of Americans categorized as obese (body mass index [BMI] >30 kg/m^2), 20% as severely obese (BMI >35), and 10% morbidly obese (BMI >40).[31]

Obesity was present in 42% of 5,700 COVID-19 patients from New York City, Long Island, and Westchester.[32] Another report from New York City of more than 4,000 patients treated at NYU Langone Medical Center from March 1 to April 2, 2020, found that if patients had a BMI greater than 40, they had a sixfold greater risk of hospitalization than normal weight COVID-patients.[33] Dr. Leora Horwitz, one of the NYU investigators, noted the independent effect that obesity has on COVID-19: "Obesity is more important for hospitalization than whether you have high blood pressure or diabetes, though these often go together, and it's more important than coronary disease or cancer or kidney disease, or even pulmonary disease. It means that as clinicians, we should be thinking a little more carefully about those patients with obesity when they come in—we should worry about them a little bit more."[34]

A systematic evaluation of studies published between January 1 and May 31, 2020, found that obesity was associated with a 39% increased risk of critical illness associated with COVID, defined as ICU admission, need for mechanical ventilation, hospice care, or death.[35] Investigators in

[30] Chen N, Zhou M, Dong X, Qu J, Gong F, Han Y, et al. Epidemiological and clinical characteristics of 99 cases of 2019 novel coronavirus pneumonia in Wuhan, China: A descriptive study. *Lancet.* February 2020;395(10223):507–513.

[31] Hales CM, Carroll MD, Fryar CD, Ogden C. Prevalence of obesity and severe obesity among adults: United States, 2017–2018. National Center for Health Statistics, Centers for Disease Control and Prevention; 2020. NCHS Data Brief No. 360.

[32] Richardson S, et al. Presenting characteristics, comorbidities, and outcomes among 5700 patients hospitalized with COVID-19 in the New York City Area. *JAMA.* April 22, 2020. 2020;323(20):2052–2059.

[33] Petrilli CM, et al. Factors associated with hospitalization and critical illness among 4,103 patients with Covid-19 disease in New York City. *medRxiv* preprint. https://doi.org/10.1101/2020.04.08.20057794.

[34] Rabin RC. Obesity linked to severe coronavirus disease, especially for younger patients. *New York Times.* April 16, 2020.

[35] Sharma A, Garg A, Rout A, Lavie CJ. Association of obesity with more critical illness in COVID-19. *Mayo Clin Proc.* 2020;95:2040–2042.

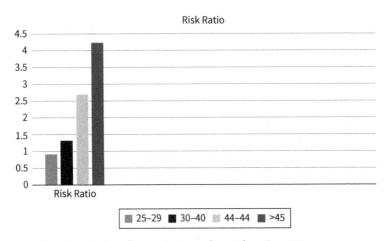

Figure 2.3. Correlation of COVID-19 Mortality with Patient BMI.
From: Tartof SY, Qian L, Hong V, et al. Obesity and mortality among patients diagnosed with COVID-19: Results from an integrated health care organization. *Ann Intern Med.* Aug 12, 2020.

France[36] and the United Kingdom[37] also found a strong correlation of obesity with COVID severity and mortality. In a study which included 7,000 COVID patients from an integrated healthcare organization in Southern California, there was a striking association between BMI and risk for death.[38] A BMI of 40–44.9 was associated with a 2.7 higher COVID death rate and BMI $\geq$45 kg/m^2 with 4.2 times higher death risk compared to normal weight patients (Figure 2.3). Dr. Roy Gulick, Chief of Infectious Diseases at Weill Cornell Medical Center, worried about younger obese patients with COVID: "If obesity does turn out to be an important risk factor for younger people, and we look at the rest of the United States—where

[36] Caussy C, Pattou F, Wallet F, Simon C, Chalopin S, Telliam C, et al. COVID Outcomes HCL Consortium and Lille COVID-Obesity Study Group. Prevalence of obesity among adult inpatients with COVID-19 in France. *Lancet Diabetes Endocrinol.* July 2020;8(7):562–564.

[37] Docherty AB, Harrison EM, Green CA, Hardwick H, Pius R, Norman L, et al. Features of 20,133 UK patients in hospital with Covid-19 using the ISARIC WHO Clinical Characterization Protocol: Prospective observational study. *BMJ.* May 22, 2020. 2020;369:m1985.

[38] Tartof SY, Qian L, Hong V, Wei R, Nadjari R, Fischer H., et al. Obesity and mortality among patients diagnosed with COVID-19: Results from an integrated health care organization. *Ann Intern Med.* Aug 12, 2020.

obesity rates are higher than in New York—that will be of great concern. We may see a lot more younger people being hospitalized."[39]

More than 77% of 17,000 patients hospitalized with COVID-19 in the United States were overweight or obese.[40] Dr. Barry Popkin, professor of nutrition at the University of North Carolina School of Public Health, cautioned, "You have more than double the likelihood of going into the hospital if you're obese and 50% more likelihood of dying. Those 2 statistics really shook me."[41] His advice to healthcare professionals was, "If they have patients who are obese or even overweight, they need to caution them to be that much more careful about COVID-19. Wear their masks. Be very careful when they're out and interacting with people outside their core family. At the same time, physicians don't do enough to talk to their patients about diet and activity and how they could improve those even with limited incomes. We need to do some of that."[42] Dr. Matthew Hutter, president of the American Society for Metabolic and Bariatric Surgery, noted, "We in the U.S. have not always identified obesity as a disease, and some people think it's a lifestyle choice. But it's not. It makes people sick, and we're realizing that now."[43]

Obesity and diabetes interfere with immune function.[44] Adipose tissue is pro-inflammatory. An excess release of cytokines causes chronic inflammation and contributes to insulin resistance. Obesity and diabetes are also associated with a hypercoagulable state.[45] Ectopic fat and COVID-19 both induce an upregulation of proinflammatory, prothrombotic, and vasoconstrictive peptide hormones. Part of obesity's adverse effect on COVID-19 patients is mechanical. Obese patients with COVID-19 hospitalized in France had a sevenfold greater risk of needing mechanical ventilation than

[39] Rabin RC. Obesity linked to severe coronavirus disease, especially for younger patients. *New York Times*. April 16, 2020.

[40] Wu K. Studies begin to untangle obesity's role in Covid-19. *The New York Times*. September 29, 2020.

[41] Abbasi J. Large meta-analysis digs into obesity's COVID-19 risks. *JAMA*. October 5, 2020. 2020;324(17):1709–1711.

[42] Abbasi J. Large meta-analysis digs into obesity's COVID-19 risks. *JAMA* October 5 2020;324(17):1709–1711.

[43] Rabin RC. Obesity linked to severe coronavirus disease, especially for younger patients. *New York Times*. April 16, 2020.

[44] Bornstein SR, Dalan R, Hopkins D, Mingrone G, Boehm BO. Endocrine and metabolic link to coronavirus infection. *Nat Rev Endocrinol*. April 2, 2020. doi: 10.1038/s41574-020-0353-9. 2020 Jun;16(6):297–298.

[45] Kimura T, Namkoong H. Susceptibility of obese population to COVID-19. *Int J Infect Dis*. October 9, 2020;101:380–381. doi: 10.1016/j.ijid.2020.10.015.

nonobese patients.[46] Abdominal adipose tissue compresses the lower part of the lungs and decreases diaphragmatic motion with subsequent decreased expiratory reserve volume, functional capacity, and respiratory system compliance. The need for mechanical ventilation in COVID-19 patients, which correlates closely with the BMI, is independent of diabetes.[47]

Both type 1 and type 2 diabetes are independent risk factors for COVID-19 morbidity and mortality. The prevalence of diabetes in COVID-19 infections has ranged from 10% to 25% in most series.[48] A study of 61 million medical records in the United Kingdom found that 30% of COVID-19 related deaths occurred in patients with diabetes.[49] Adjusted for multiple variables, the odds ratio for in-hospital COVID-related death was 3.5 in those with type 1 diabetes and 2.0 for those with type 2 diabetes. A study in China found that the CFR of COVID-19 patients with type 2 diabetes was three times greater than those without diabetes.[50] Fasting blood sugar was an independent predictor of mortality in COVID-19 patients who did not have a previous diagnosis of diabetes.[51]

Long-Term Care Facilities

As of January 2, 2021, about 40% of the COVID-19 deaths in the United States had been from long-term care facilities (LTCFs), although less than 1% of the population resides in LTCFs.[52] LTCFs include nursing homes, skilled

---

[46] Simonnet A, et al. High prevalence of obesity in severe respiratory syndrome coronavirus-2 (SARS-CoV-2) requiring invasive mechanical ventilation. *Obesity*. April 9, 2020.

[47] Simonnet A, et al. High prevalence of obesity in severe respiratory syndrome coronavirus-2 (SARS-CoV19) requiring invasive mechanical ventilation. *Obesity*. April 9, 2020.

[48] Singh AK, Gupta R, Ghosh A. Misra A. Diabetes in COVID-19: Prevalence, pathophysiology, prognosis and practical considerations. *Diab & Met Syn: Clin Res & Rev*. 2020;14:303–310. https://doi.org/10.1016/j.dsx.2020.04.004.

[49] Barron E, Bakhai C, Kar P, Weaver A, Bradley D, Ismail H, et al. Associations of type 1 and type 2 diabetes with COVID-19-related mortality in England: A whole-population study. *Lancet Diabetes & Endo*. August 13, 2020. doi: 10.1016/S2213-8587(20)30272-2.

[50] Wu C, et al. Risk factors associated with acute respiratory distress syndrome and death in patients with coronavirus disease 2019 pneumonia in Wuhan, China. *JAMA Intern Med*. March 13, 2020;180(7):934–943.

[51] Wang S, Ma P, Zhang S, Song S, Wang Z, Ma Y, et al. Fasting blood glucose at admission is an independent predictor for 28-day mortality in patients with COVID-19 without previous diagnosis of diabetes: A multi-centre retrospective study. *Diabetologia*. July 10, 2020. doi: 10.1007/s00125-020-05209-1.

[52] Covid in the U.S.: Latest map and case count. *The New York Times*. October 30, 2020.

nursing facilities, retirement homes, assisted-living facilities, and residential care homes. In 2020, there had been more than 1 million cases of COVID-19 in residents and staff of US LTCFs, with 133,000 deaths. Approximately 1 million adults live in the 25,000 LTCFs in the United States and most have chronic medical conditions as well as problems with mobility and cognition.[53] About 44% of American men and 58% of women over age 65 will use nursing homes at some time in their lives.[54]

During the first few months of the pandemic, the overall COVID-19 CFR for residents of US LTCFs was 33%.[55] In the United Kingdom, there were three times as many deaths in LTCFs between March 2 and June 12 of 2020 compared to the previous year.[56] Two-thirds of those were directly related to COVID-19. In Belgium from March to May, more than 60% of COVID-related deaths occurred in the LTCF population.[57] In Scotland, residence in an LTCF was associated with a twenty-one-fold increased rate of severe COVID, dwarfing other risk factors, such as age, race, and comorbidity.[58] About 40%–50% of COVID-related deaths in the United States, France, Sweden, the United Kingdom, and Germany were in LTCFs.[59] In Canada, mortality incidence for a resident aged 70 or older of an LTCF was 13 times higher than that of a same-age resident in the general population.[60] Mortality

[53] The COVID Tracking Project. *The Atlantic.* Accessed December 30, 2020. https://www.theatlantic.com/science/

[54] Barnett ML, Hu L, Martin T, Grabowski DC. Mortality, admissions, and patient census at SNFs in 3 US cities during the COVID-19 pandemic. *JAMA.* August4;324:507.

[55] Centers for Medicare & Medicaid Services. Long-term care facility reporting on COVID-19. 2020. Accessed June 5, 2020. https://www.cms.gov/files/document/covid-nursing-home-reporting-numbers-5-31-20.pdf.

[56] BBC News. Coronavirus: Almost 30,000 excess care homes deaths. July 3, 2020.

[57] Molenberghs G, Faes C, Aerts J, Theeten H, Devleesschauwer B, Bustos Sierra N, et al. Belgian Covid-19 mortality, excess deaths, number of deaths per million, and infection fatality rates (8 March–9 May 2020). *medRxiv.* June 20, 2020. https://doi.org/10.1101/2020.06.20.20136234

[58] McKeigue PM, Weir A, Bishop J, McGurnaghan SJ, Kennedy S, McAllister D, et al. Rapid epidemiological analysis of comorbidities and treatments as risk factors for COVID-19 in Scotland (REACT-SCOT): A population-based case-control study. *PLoS Med.* October 20, 2020;17(10):e1003374. doi: 10.1371/journal.pmed.1003374.

[59] Denyer S, Kashiwagi A. Japan has the world's oldest population. Yet it dodged a coronavirus crisis at elder-care facilities. *The Washington Post.* August 30, 2020.

[60] Fisman DN, Bogoch I, Lapointe-Shaw L, McCready J, Tuite AR. Risk factors associated with mortality among residents with coronavirus disease (COVID-19) in long-term care facilities in Ontario, Canada. *JAMA Network Open.* 2020;3(7):e2015957. doi:10.1001/jamanetworkopen.2020.15957.

risk factors for COVID patients in LTCFs included age, male sex, and impaired physical or cognitive function.[61] The pandemic gained attention in the United States in early April after a single case was identified and then followed closely at a skilled nursing facility in Kirkland, Washington.[62] Within 3 weeks, 64% of that facility had tested positive and one-quarter of the patients had died. In the early phases of the pandemic, hospitals were relying on LTCFs to relieve their inpatient burden from infected patients. Patients who had recovered from COVID and were deemed stable were quickly transferred to LTCFs when home care was not possible or available. Governor Andrew Cuomo of New York described nursing homes as a "feeding frenzy for this virus . . . but they had to accept the patients—but only, if they could do so safely. Homes unable to comply should transfer them to other facilities or notify the state Health Department."[63]

With fragile older people living in close contact, LTCFs have always been vulnerable to nosocomial infections. These hazards were greatly magnified with the pandemic. Dr. Sunil Parikh, an infectious disease specialist at Yale School of Medicine, described the influx of patients from LTCFs: "It is only Saturday afternoon and our emergency department has already seen the fourth patient with Covid-19 from one of the local nursing homes this weekend. She was fine just a few days ago; now she is disoriented and can't catch her breath. At age 75 and with other chronic conditions, should we put her on an experimental therapy? A few hours later, an ambulance brings a patient from a different nursing home, one that already has 21 residents with Covid-19 cases, three of whom died in the past week. He is 87 years old, has severe heart disease, is unresponsive, and no family member is reachable. He needs to be placed on a ventilator in order to survive, but once on the machine, his chance of getting off it alive is not great . . . we've missed another important mark by not focusing on residents in long-term care facilities, as

[61] Panagiotou OA, Kosar CM, White EM, Bantis LE, Yang X, Santostefano CM, et al. Risk factors associated with all-cause mortality in nursing home residents with COVID-19. *JAMA Intern Med.* January 4, 2021; doi: 10.1001/jamainternmed.2020.7968.

[62] McMichael TM, Currie DW, Clark S, Pogosjans S, Kay M, Schwartz NG, et al. Epidemiology of Covid-19 in a long-term care facility in King County, Washington. *N Engl J Med.* May 21, 2020;382:2005–2011. doi: 10.1056/NEJMoa2005412.

[63] Kim Barker and Amy Julia Harris. "Playing Russian Roulette": Nursing homes told to take the infected. *New York Times.* April 24, 2020.

they make up the largest proportion of Covid-19 cases that are hitting our hospitals, requiring ventilation, and succumbing to the virus."[64]

In addition to the increased COVID-19-related mortality in residents of LTCFs, there was a profound adverse effect from their enforced social isolation. State and local officials banned visitors and any nonessential healthcare personnel and canceled communal activities within the LTCFs. Goldie Albertson, a 79-year-old nursing home resident, complained, "I remember when the polio came out, it wasn't like this. We weren't locked up in our homes. We can't leave the building right now with this crazy virus. It's the same way, all the time. It is hard. It's hard when you can't go anywhere."[65] Dr. Ken Covinsky, a geriatrician at the University of California, San Francisco, worried about such isolation: "It's not just touchy-feely stuff. Isolation is a real risk. We have restricted something that's pretty essential. We need to move away from thinking of visitors to old people as optional."[66] Dr. Dallas Nelson, the medical director of two nursing homes in Rochester, New York, said, "We now have a handful of people we think have actually died because they've been in isolation and haven't had any contact at all with their families. It's accelerating their dementia and failure to thrive. The antidote is unequivocally to open up as much as possible, in every way possible, as soon as possible, while still following the rules. With masks we should be letting patients eat in congregant dining, do activities with appropriate distance and, most importantly, visit with family and caregivers."[67]

LTCFs everywhere were overlooked or simply ignored by governments and suffered from inadequate personal protective equipment (PPE), limited testing, and limited access to critical care facilities. According to Alice Bonner, of the Institute for Healthcare Improvement, healthcare workers at LTCFs "are making $12 or $13 an hour. They can barely support themselves and their families. Some of them are working in nursing homes during the day, then assisted living in the evening and home health at night."[68]

---

[64] Parikh S. Nursing homes, veterans' homes are national epicenters of Covid-19. *STAT.* May 8, 2020.

[65] Ross E, Nierenberg A. It's hard when you can't go anywhere: Life inside an assisted living facility. *New York Times.* May 9, 2020.

[66] Parikh S. Nursing homes, veterans' homes are national epicenters of Covid-19. *STAT.* May 8, 2020.

[67] Abbasi J. "Abandoned" nursing homes continue to face critical supply and staff shortages as COVID-19 toll has mounted. *JAMA.* June 11, 2020.

[68] Kim ET. This is why nursing homes failed so badly. *The New York Times.* December 31, 2020.

Belgium's public health response to COVID in nursing homes was particularly outrageous. Even after the World Health Organization (WHO) declared that it was essential to create plans to protect LTCFs, a spokesperson for Belgium said, "The risk of infection is very low now." LTCFs weren't given aid or priority testing and their residents were denied hospital admissions.[69] Dr. Michel Hanset, a physician in Brussels, said, "The decision not to accept residents in hospitals really shocked me."[70] LTCFs in the United States were also "forcing people out," and, according to a long-term New Jersey ombudsman, "It felt opportunistic, where some homes were basically seizing the moment when everyone is looking the other way to move people out."[71]

LTCF morbidity and mortality from COVID-19 correlated with the pre-existing quality of the LTCF, which was generally poor well before the pandemic. According to a 2014 report, one-third of Medicare LTCF residents suffered harm within 2 weeks of entry, and there were 3 million infections yearly at US LTCFs.[72] Across eight states, LTCFs with increased nurse staffing had fewer COVID cases.[73] A study of 618 Canadian LTCFs found a correlation of resident crowding with COVID-19 infections and mortality.[74] Modeling demonstrated that converting all four-bedroom units to two-bedrooms would have averted 20% of infections and deaths.

About 70% of LTCFs are owned by for-profit companies, including private investment firms, and their quality ratings are generally below those of non-profit LTCFs.[75] These for-profit companies grabbed the lion's share of pandemic relief under the CARES Act, including a dozen companies accused of Medicare fraud that received more than $300 million.[76] David Grabowski,

[69] Stevis-Gridneff M, Apuzzo M, Pronczuk M. When COVID-19 hit, many elderly were left to die. *The New York Times*. August 8, 2020.

[70] Stevis-Gridneff M, Apuzzo M, Pronczuk M. When COVID-19 hit, many elderly were left to die. *The New York Times*. August 8, 2020.

[71] Silver-Greenberg J, Harris AJ. "They just dumped him like trash": Nursing homes evict vulnerable residents. *The New York Times*. June 21, 2020.

[72] Mollot R. Nursing homes were a disaster waiting to happen. *The New York Times*. April 28, 2020.

[73] Figueroa JF, Wadhera RK, Papanicolos I, Riley K, Zheng J, Orav EJ, et al. Association of nursing home ratings on health inspections, quality of care, and nurse staffing with COVID-19 cases. *JAMA*. August 10, 2020;324(11):1103–1105. doi:10.1001/jama.2020.14709.

[74] Brown KA, Jones A, Daneman N, Chan AK, Schwartz KL, Garber GE, et al. Association between nursing home crowding and COVID-19 infection and mortality in Ontario, Canada. *JAMA Int Med*. November 9, 2021;181(2):229–236. doi:10.1001/jamainternmed.2020.6466.

[75] Goldstein M, Silver-Greenberg J, Gebeloff R. Push for profits left nursing homes struggling to provide care. *The New York Times*. May 7, 2020.

[76] Kim ET. This is why nursing homes failed so badly. *The New York Times*. December 31, 2020.

professor of healthcare policy at Harvard Medical School, noted, "With this huge health crisis and economic downturn, we are all of a sudden seeing how risky it is to have the ownership split between the real estate side that has the most valuable asset and the operator, who is left with much less."[77]

As in the general population, CFRs were higher at LTCFs with an increased percentage of Black and Hispanic residents. Dr. David Gifford, chief medical officer for the American Health Care Association, said, "Typically, what occurs in the general population is mirrored in long-term care facilities."[78] One study found that the death rate was more than 20% higher in majority-Black facilities compared with majority-White facilities and death rates increased as the proportion of Black residents increased.[79] LTCFs with a significant portion of Black and Latino residents were twice as likely to have COVID infections as those with largely White residents.[80] In New York, 84% of LTCFs with at least 25% Black and Latino population reported COVID-19 infections compared to 33% with less than 5% Black and Latino populations.[81]

Widespread lack of PPE in LTCFs persisted throughout 2020. A LTCF that needed 1,400 hospital gowns weekly for its staff received a shipment of 432 in May 2020.[82] Lori Smetanka, executive director of the National Consumer Voice for Quality Long-Term Care, said, "Every day we hear about the critical needs for protective personal equipment for staff, for testing for residents, and until those things are prioritized for long-term care facilities, I think we're not at the point where we're going to see this getting under control."[83]

The testing deficiencies throughout the United States were especially dangerous for residents and staff at LTCFs. It took until May 18 for the Centers for Medicare and Medicaid to recommend regular universal testing for all nursing home staff and residents—namely that all residents should be

[77] Goldstein M, Silver-Greenberg J, Gebeloff R. Push for profits left nursing homes struggling to provide care. *The New York Times*. May 7, 2020.

[78] Gebeloff R, Ivory D, Richtel M, Smith M, Yourish K, Dance S, et al. The striking racial divide in how covid-19 has hit nursing homes. *The New York Times*. September 10, 2020.

[79] King S, Jacobs J. Near birthplace of Martin Luther King Jr., a predominantly Black nursing home tries to heal outbreak. *The Washington Post*. September 9, 2020.

[80] Gebeloff R, Ivory D, Richtel M, Smith M, Yourish K, Dance S, et al. The striking racial divide in how Covid-19 has hit nursing homes. *The New York Times*. September 10, 2020.

[81] Gebeloff R, Ivory D, Richtel M, Smith M, Yourish K, Dance S, et al. The striking racial divide in how Covid-19 has hit nursing homes. *The New York Times*. September 10, 2020.

[82] Abbasi J. "Abandoned" nursing homes continue to face critical supply and staff shortages as COVID-19 toll has mounted. *JAMA*. June 11, 2020.

[83] Abbasi J. "Abandoned" nursing homes continue to face critical supply and staff shortages as COVID-19 toll has mounted. *JAMA*. June 11, 2020.

retested if anyone develops COVID-19 symptoms or tests positive for the virus and then every resident retested weekly until all test negative.[84]

The spike in COVID cases nationally in the fall of 2020 once again hit LTCFs the hardest, as was noted by geriatrician Dr. Shannon Tapia: "This is much, much worse than the spring. Covid is going crazy in Colorado right now. It just happens so fast. There's no time to send them back. Systematically, it makes me feel like I'm failing. The last eight months almost broke me."[85]

Gender

As of December 21, 2020, 52% of COVID-19 cases in the United States had been in females but 54% of deaths were in males and the coronavirus had killed almost 17,000 more American men than women.[86] In a global analysis of more than 3 million cases of COVID-19, there was no difference in proportion of males and females with confirmed infection, but males had almost three times the odds of ICU admission and a greater mortality risk.[87] Dr. Franck Mauvais-Jarvis, who does research on gender differences in chronic diseases, said, "If you look at the data across the world, there are as many men as women that are infected. It's just the severity of disease that is stronger in most populations in men."[88]

The increased male mortality rate has been attributed to biologic and social factors. Men do have a higher comorbidity prevalence than females, but that alone could not explain the gender differences in COVID-19 mortality.[89] Women have a stronger immune response than men. Estrogens promote

[84] Abbasi J. "Abandoned" nursing homes continue to face critical supply and staff shortages as COVID-19 toll has mounted. *JAMA*. June 11, 2020.

[85] Wu K. Covid combat fatigue: I would come home with tears in my eyes. *The New York Times*. November 25, 2020.

[86] CDC COVID Data tracker. Accessed December 21, 2020.

[87] Peckham H, de Gruiter NM, Raine C, Radziszewska A, Ciurtin C, Wedderburn LR, et al. Male sex identified by global meta-analysis as a risk factor for death and ITU admission. *Nature Communications*. December 9, 2020.

[88] Guarino B. Why the coronavirus is killing more men than women. *The Washington Post*. October 17, 2020.

[89] Alkhouli M, Nanjundappa A, Annie F, Bates MC, Bhatt DL. Sex differences in case fatality rate of COVID-19: Insights from a multinational registry. *Mayo Clin Proc*. August 2020;95(8):1613–1620. doi: 10.1016/j.mayocp.2020.05.014.

innate and adaptive immunity, with increased ability to clear infections and greater vaccine efficacy. Women have a higher incidence of autoimmune diseases, such as systemic lupus erythematosus and rheumatoid arthritis, but they are more capable of fighting off infections.[90] T cell and B cell reactivity to SARS-Cov-2 was weaker in men, which was also blunted with aging, noting that "the reduction in NK cell–activating receptors and up-regulation of negative regulators of immune effector function—and resultant throttling of effector function—is consistent with a more severe manifestation of COVID-19 in males."[91] A blunted T cell response with age was associated with poor outcomes in males but not in females with COVID-19 infection.[92] Men with severe COVID-19 infection compared to women more often had autoantibodies directed against interferon.[93]

Social and behavioral gender differences also impact the sex discrepancies in COVID-19 fatalities. Women have been more likely to treat health risks seriously and follow public health advice, whereas occupation risks are greater in men.[94] The increase death rate in men decreases when looking at women working full-time. Sarah Hawkes, a professor of global public health at University College, London, said, "The more you have women participating in the workforce, the smaller your sex difference becomes. That lines up with gender inequalities—men are more likely to work in environments where they are exposed to air pollution and other harms." When women start to enter those traditionally masculine spaces, she said, it "turns out, women can get as sick as men."[95] As with age, the gender differences in response to COVID-19 must be factored in as vaccine studies progress.

[90] vom Steeg LG, Klein SL. SeXX Matters in Infectious Disease Pathogenesis. *PloS Pathog.* February 2016;12(2):e1005374. pmid:26891052.

[91] Lieberman NAP, Peddu V, Xie H, Shrestha L, Huang M- L, Mears MC, et al. In vivo antiviral host transcriptional response to SARS-CoV-2 by viral load, sex, and age. *PLoS Biol.* September 8, 2020.

[92] Takahashi T, Ellingson MK, Iwasaki A. Sex differences in immune responses that underlie COVID-19 disease outcomes. *Nature.* August 26, 2020. 2020;588:315–320. https://doi.org/10.1038/s41586-020-2700-3.

[93] Bastard P, Rosen LB, Zhang Q, Michailidis E, Hoffman H- H, Zhang Y, et al. Autoantibodies against type I IFNs in patients with life-threatening COVID-19. *Science.* October 23, 2020;370(6515):eabd4585. doi 10.1126/science.abd4585.

[94] Guarino B. Why the coronavirus is killing more men than women. *The Washington Post.* October 17, 2020.

[95] Guarino B. Why the coronavirus is killing more men than women. *The Washington Post.* October 17, 2020.

Race and Ethnicity

In the United States, Blacks and Hispanics, compared to non-Hispanic Whites, have a two-to-three-times higher rate of COVID-19 infection, and a two-to-three-times higher rate of hospitalization and death.[96] US deaths per 100,000 as of mid-December 2020 were much higher for Hispanic, Native Americans, and Black/African Americans than for Asian or White Americans (Figure 2.4).[97] Dr. Lisa Cooper, the Director of the Johns Hopkins Center for Health Equity, noted, "While Black Americans represent only about 13% of the population in the states reporting racial/ethnic information, they account for about 34% of total Covid-19 deaths in those states."[98] The racial inequities are even more striking in young people. More than a quarter of deaths in Latino patients with COVID infections were younger than age 60 compared to 6% in White patients.[98] Dr. David Ansell, the Director of Community Health Equity at Rush University Medical Center in Chicago, said, "An epidemic shows in a short period of time what's been going on for hundreds of years."[99]

Racial inequities are not unique to the United States. Death rates from COVID in the United Kingdom were significantly higher for Black patients, with a standardized mortality ratio (SMR) of 3.2.[100] The fatality rate of COVID-19 patients of Black African descent in English hospitals was 3.5 times that of White British patients.[101]

These striking differences in rates of infection and fatality are related to structural inequities in minority communities. Minority groups are overrepresented in lower income brackets, more likely to have jobs on the

[96] Mackey K, Ayers CK, Kondo KK, Saha S, Advani SM, Young S, et al. Racial and ethnic disparities in COVID-19-related infections, hospitalizations and deaths. *Ann Intern Med.* December 1, 2020. doi: 10.7326/M20-6306.

[97] The COVID Tracking Project. *The Atlantic.* Accessed December 21, 2020.

[98] Oppel Jr RA, Gebeloff R, Lai KKR, Wright W, Smith M. The fullest look yet at racial inequity of coronavirus. *The New York Times.* July 5, 2020.

[99] Wezerek G. Racism's hidden toll. *The New York Times.* August 11, 2020.

[100] Aldridge, et al. Black, Asian and Minority Ethnic groups in England are at increased risk of death from COVID-19: Indirect standardisation of NHS mortality data. *Wellcome Open Res.* May 5, 2020. https://www.ncbi.nlm.nih.gov/pmc/articles/PMC7317462/. Accessed May 5, 2020.

[101] Otu A, Ahinkorah BO, Ameyaw EK, Seidu A-A, Yaya S. One country, two crises: What Covid-19 reveals about health inequalities among BAME communities in the United Kingdom and the sustainability of its health system? *Int J Equity Health* 2020;19(1):189. doi: 10.1186/s12939-020-01307-z.

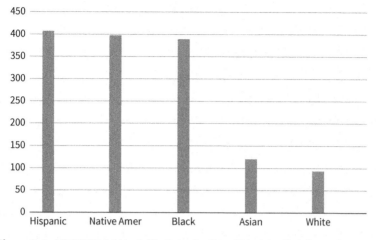

Figure 2.4. US COVID-19 Mortality Rates by Race/Ethnicity. Death rates per 100,000 cases.
From: The COVID Tracking Project. *The Atlantic.* Accessed December 21, 2020.

front line, experience more crowded conditions and become exposed to greater air pollution with subsequent increased rates of asthma. There are greater rates of diabetes, obesity, hypertension, and heart disease in Black and Hispanic Americans, each closely linked to socioeconomic factors with subsequent poor health outcomes.[102] Dr. Mary Bassett, the Director of the FXB Center for Health and Human Rights at Harvard University, commented that the sole focus on comorbidities "makes me angry, because this really is about who still has to leave their home to work, who has to leave a crowded apartment, get on crowded transport, and go to a crowded workplace, and we just haven't acknowledged that those of us who have the privilege of continuing to work from our homes aren't facing those risks."[103]

Black mothers in the United States die at four times the rate of White mothers, and their infant mortality rate is twice as high.[104] A Black patient on average receives $1,800 less per year on medical care compared to a White

[102] Garibaldi BT, Fiksel J, Muschelli J, Robinson ML, Rouhizadeh M, Perin J, et al. Patient trajectories among persons hospitalized with COVID-19. *Ann Intern Med.* September 22, 2020. https://doi.org/10.7326/M20-3905.
[103] Oppel Jr RA, Gebeloff R, Lai KKR, Wright W, Smith M. The fullest look yet at racial inequity of coronavirus. *The New York Times.* July 5, 2020.
[104] Pearl R. Coronavirus deaths show how little black lives matter in American healthcare. *Forbes.* July 15, 2020.

person with the same health issues. Blacks are 60% more likely not to have health insurance than Whites.[105]

Hospitals in Black communities received less COVID-19 funding than their White counterparts despite a greater burden of infections.[106] Dr. Michele Evans has stated that "The disproportionate effects of the COVID-19 pandemic on African Americans, Latinx Americans, and Native Americans is not unforeseen. Inequities in health, healthcare access, and quality of care are ingrained in the US healthcare system. Medical mistrust, limited healthcare access, and other factors lead to late diagnosis and suboptimal management of infectious diseases among vulnerable minority populations. Now, engulfed in the catastrophic pandemic maelstrom, we are reckoning with a deadly triad—health disparities, health inequity, and unequal health care access—quantified in a daily body count."[107]

[105] Greenhouse S. The coronavirus pandemic has intensified systemic economic racism against black Americans. *The New Yorker.* July 30, 2020.

[106] Ross C. Study finds racial bias in the government's formula for distributing Covid-19 aid to hospitals. *STAT.* August 7, 2020.

[107] Evans MK. Covid's color line-infectious disease, inequity, and racial justice. *N Engl J Med.* July 30, 2020. 2020;383:408–410. doi: 10.1056/NEJMp2019445.

3

Impact on Healthcare Workers and Hospitals

Healthcare Workers

Early during the pandemic, hospitals and healthcare workers (HCWs) were overwhelmed with COVID patients. There was an urgent need to increase ICU beds and staffing, as well as respiratory therapy, triage, and isolation and containment units. Dr. Danielle Ofri described the dramatic changes in physicians' job descriptions early on in the pandemic: "Attending physicians are being pulled from everywhere—clinic, cardiology, G.I., rheumatology, retirement. Senior residents from urology, orthopedics, surgery, and ophthalmology have been drafted to be interns on the medicine service. I spend the morning on the wards with a colleague who normally practices psychiatry and addiction medicine. We're rounding with a dermatology resident, a senior orthopedic resident, and a hastily graduated medical student all acting as medicine interns, plus one regular medical resident and a trio of imported nurse practitioners with accents ranging from deep Southern drawl to Midwestern flat—the typical pastiche that constitutes a medical team these days. The staffing schedule looks like a NASA flowchart for the moon landing. Every day, the rules of engagement reshuffle."[1]

More than 20,000 HCWs, including 4,000 nurses from all over the United States, volunteered for hazard duty in New York during the surge of COVID cases in March and April. Heather Smith, a nurse from a small island off the coast of North Carolina working at Elmhurst Hospital Center in Queens, worried, "Every day you go in and you're like, 'Can I do this for one more day? Why did I wake up?'" Tamara Williams, a 40-year-old nurse from Dallas, said, "I have never seen patients so sick before. And dying, despite

---

[1] Ofri D. The public has been forgiving. But hospitals got some things wrong. *The New York Times*. May 22, 2020. Accessed May 22, 2020. https://www.newyorktimes.com/

everything that we're doing."[2] Describing her new coworkers, "I see them crying over this person they worked with for so long, and I'm just imagining my own people back home."[3]

Despite being the wealthiest nation in the world, the United States fell woefully short in supplying personal protective equipment (PPE) for HCWs and patients. Adequate supply of masks, gowns and gloves, and medical devices, especially supplemental oxygen and ventilators, quickly ran dry.[4] N95 respirators, designed for single use, were now being used for days on end or were simply unavailable. In early March, Dr. Stephen Anderson, who had worked in a Seattle emergency room for more than 35 years, said he was down to wearing one surgical mask per shift, cleaning the mask each time he saw a new patient. "Those are supposed to be disposable. That may sound just like a nuisance, but when you're potentially touching something that has the virus that could kill you on it, and you're doing it 25 times a shift, it's kind of nerve-racking. Most physicians have never seen this level of angst and anxiety in their careers. Now that we see front-line providers that are on ventilators, it is really driving it home. I am sort of a pariah in my family. I am dipping myself into the swamp every day." A resident physician in Boston said, "We get one per shift, per day . . . I had a surgical mask and a face shield I had been cleaning and reusing for a month."[5] Dr. Hooman Kamel, who worked in one of the first ICUs dedicated entirely to patients with COVID-19 but ran low on PPE, commented, "Everyone at my place can get at least one N95, which they can then reuse. They just get one. It's not ideal. I am wearing a mask at all times, which is pretty terrible. I think the smell of surgical masks is going to be seared in my brain for life."[6] Supply of surgical gowns became so low that some medical personnel began wearing rain ponchos and makeshift garbage bags for protection.

PPE shortages popped up again with each surge of the pandemic. A survey of 20,000 nurses in August 2020 found that 68% were reusing N95 masks,

[2] Gross J. Hundreds of miles from home, nurses fight coronavirus on New York's front lines. *The New York Times*. April 28, 2020.

[3] Gross J. Hundreds of miles from home, nurses fight coronavirus on New York's front lines. *The New York Times*. April 28, 2020.

[4] Chou R, Dana T, Buckley DJ, Selph S, Fu R, Totten AM. Epidemiology of and risk factors for coronavirus infection in health care workers: A living rapid review. July 21 2020;173(2):120–136. *Ann Intern Med* May 5, 2020.

[5] Baird R. How doctors on the front lines are confronting the uncertainties of COVID-19. *The New Yorker*. April 5, 2020.

[6] Baird R. Doctors on the front lines, *The New Yorker*. April 5, 2020.

often for more than 5 days.[7] Nurses with critical-care training were in short supply throughout the country. An ICU nurse was working six 12-hour shifts weekly and said, "We are not OK. People think a nurse is a nurse is a nurse, but they are just as specialized as doctors."[8]

The three chief residents at one of the largest internal medicine programs in the United States described the relentless uncertainty. "Our residents had a constant stream of questions, to which we could often only provide unsatisfying answers. The manner in which residents reacted to the loss of their educational experience, the loss of their personal lives, and the loss of their patients and loved ones could never be fairly judged or categorized. How is one supposed to deal with such profound loss during a vulnerable time in one's career and life? We did not know. However, as we navigated the complexities of the pandemic, we eventually found ourselves relying on one phrase: Thank you for your flexibility during these unprecedented times."[9]

Redeployment of physicians and nurses was very stressful. Clinicians asked, "How much choice will I have in where I'm deployed," and hospital leaders attempted to reassure them that they would not be asked to do anything they weren't comfortable with and redeploy them not more than "one degree of separation from their customary role."[10] Dr. Rahul Sharma, the Emergency Physician-in-Chief at New York-Presbyterian/Weill Cornell Medical Center, described staff redeployment: "One of the biggest challenges was the trepidation some providers had. You've never trained in emergency medicine, and now you are asked to go to an emergency department, which is busy during a pandemic. It could be scary. We wanted to make sure that they felt part of the team. Also, clinically, we wanted to make sure that they were given appropriate training. A lot of them had to be trained, but this all happened in the course of 1 to 2 weeks. We've learned and continue to learn a great deal from this Covid epidemic. One thing I'm certain of is that we will have to rethink the way we do things regarding workflows and processes. From an institutional standpoint, departments will no longer be able to be

[7] American Nurses Association. Update on nurses and PPE. www.nursingworld.org. ANA Enterprise. Accessed October 23, 2020.

[8] Nuila R. To fight the coronavirus, you need an army. *The New Yorker.* July 17, 2020.

[9] Ou A, Torres CL, Rufin M. Thank you for your flexibility during these unprecedented times. *JAMA Intern Med.* 2020;180(10):1278–1279. doi:10.1001/jamainternmed.2020.3020.

[10] Haas S, Smith RE. As clinicians are redeployed for Covid-19, onboarding takes on extra importance. *STAT.* August 6, 2020.

siloed and will have to lean on each other and call upon each other much more frequently and much more substantially."[11]

The Department of Medicine at the Keck School of Medicine at the University of Southern California surveyed its faculty confidentially regarding individual willingness and risk potential for critical care.[12] Those willing and able to participate in "surge duty" were given positions that optimally matched their background and then received structured training from intensivists and hospitalists. At New York City hospitals, staff deployed to the frontline were given weekly orientation sessions, supplemented by detailed COVID-care manuals.[13] Attending physicians, fellows, and residents received a refresher course on ventilator management, pressor use, line placement, and point-of-care ultrasound. Senior medical students who had completed their coursework were accredited as residents. Students in clerkships worked online to field family queries and review clinical and research data.

Doctors, nurses, and all frontline workers were faced with unprecedented physical and emotional trauma and had to deal with potential personal harm, not only to themselves but also to their families. Dr. Stephanie Taylor recalled, "In the early weeks of the pandemic, there was so much fear at the hospital—fear that I would not have enough personal protective equipment (PPE), fear that even adequate PPE would not prevent transmission of the virus during high-risk encounters, fear that I did not know how to help my patients, fear that I would have to choose who to help and who to deny lifesaving therapy. There was incalculable fear at home, too—fear that my husband or I might bring home severe acute respiratory syndrome and endanger our children or each other, fear that my children would suffer psychological consequences from isolation or remote education, fear that we might not have reliable access to food, basic supplies, or other necessities."[14]

[11] Sharma R, Seth Mohta N. Pivoting quickly: Redesigning ED care in New York City to take on Covid-19. *N Engl J Med.* April 29, 2020. https://catalyst.nejm.org/doi/full/10.1056/CAT.20.0196. Accessed May 5, 2021.

[12] Kumar SI, Borok Z. Filling the bench: Faculty surge deployment in response to the Covid-19 pandemic. *N Engl J Med.* October 29, 2020. https://catalyst.nejm.org/doi/full/10.1056/CAT.20.0511. Accessed May 5, 2021.

[13] Schaye VE, Reich JA, Bosworth BP, Stern DT, Volpicelli F, Shapiro NM, et al. Collaborating across private, public, community, and federal hospital systems: Lessons learned from the Covid-19 pandemic response in NYC. *N Engl J Med.* November–December 2020 doi:10.1056/CAT.20.0343.

[14] Taylor S. Shear forces. *JAMA.* October 28, 2020;324(19):1943–1944. doi:10.1001/jama.2020.21746.

Physicians portrayed differing phases of emotional distress during COVID. Dr. Jonathan Kochav, a cardiology fellow in New York, said that early on in his treating COVID patients, "Dealing with family members was particularly emotional. I saw my fears coming true in what they were experiencing. I could so easily project myself into their position. I felt disconnected. I'm not sure if it's because I overinvested earlier and was just emotionally spent, or because every day was an endless stream of the same thing. But I went from seeing every patient as my mom, my dad, my wife, to seeing every patient as a lab value and ventilator setting."[15] A paramedic said that he and his crew felt overwhelmed. "The virus scares the hell out of our guys. And now, when they go home to decompress, instead, they and their spouses are home schooling. The spouse has lost a job, and is at wit's end. The kids are screaming. Let me tell you: The tension level in the crews is through the roof."[16]

Hospital no-visitor policies contributed to the loneliness HCWs faced during the pandemic, as explained by Dr. Dhruv Khullar. "In the I.C.U., clinicians are used to caring for patients who arc intubated, sedated, or simply too ill to speak. That challenge, though, is usually offset by the richness of their interactions with family. Now we see only oxygen tubes and heart monitors; we hear only labored breaths and bedside alarms. There are no families whispering well wishes or holding patients' hands. Watching someone suffer alone is its own form of punishment. Now many doctors treating the coronavirus find that their patients' isolation is paired with their own. Some are socially distancing from their own families—sleeping in hotel rooms near the hospital to avoid exposing their households to the virus. Others go home, but eat and sleep separately, in the basement or a garage. As weeks pass away from friends and family, we find ourselves leaning more on each other—providing not just clinical care to our patients but emotional support to our colleagues."[17] Dr. Richard Leiter led a palliative care team within a Boston hospital's ICU and described, "We spoke to countless families over the phone and by Zoom calls to tell them their loved ones were critically ill, getting sicker, and eventually, dying. When the prognosis seemed dire,

[15] Khullar D. The emotional evolution of coronavirus doctors and patients. *The New Yorker.* July 7, 2020.
[16] Hoffman J. "I can't turn my brain off": PTSD and burnout threaten medical workers. *The New York Times.* May 16, 2020.
[17] Khullar D. "A disembodied voice": The loneliness and solidarity of treating the coronavirus in New York. *The New Yorker.* April 8, 2020.

we recommended transitioning to comfort focused care. And in patients' final hours and days, we held iPads at their bedsides so that family members around the world could say goodbye. Over time, perhaps we'll uncover the toll Covid-19 has taken on clinicians."[18]

The unprecedented stress associated with the pandemic resulted in a marked increase in mental health problems in HCWs throughout the world. HCW prevalence of depression, anxiety, and posttraumatic stress disorder (PTSD) during the pandemic ranged from 30% to 70% and were especially prominent in physicians and nurses on the frontline.[19] More than 50% of Chinese HCWs reported depressed mood during the early phase of COVID-19,[20] and there was a sharp rise in depression and anxiety in first-year Chinese medical residents during the pandemic.[21] In an April survey of 1,000 HCWs in New York, 58% screened positive for depression and 33% for anxiety (Figure 3.1).[22] Acute stress with symptoms of PTSD were found in 65% of nurses, 55% of residents and fellows, and 40% of attending physicians. HCWs who had close contact with infected patients—including HCWs in emergency departments, ICUs, and ambulance services—were more likely to suffer mental health distress.[23] Symptoms of PTSD were found in 30% of 1,773 HCWs in Norway during the pandemic and the symptoms correlated with amount of direct exposure to patients with COVID-19.[24]

Dr. Srijan Sen, a professor of psychiatry at the University of Michigan, who had been treating physicians during the pandemic, said, "We saw a

[18] Leiter RE. Reentry. *N Engl J Med.* October 14, 2020. 2020;383:e141. doi: 10.1056/NEJMp2027447.

[19] Braquehais MD, Vargas-Caceres S, Gomez-Duran E, Nieva G, Valero S, Casas M, et al. The impact of the COVID-19 pandemic on the mental health of healthcare professionals. *QJM.* July 1, 2020. doi10.1093/qjmed/hcaa207.

[20] Lai J, Ma S, Wang Y. Factors associated with mental health outcomes among health care workers exposed to coronavirus disease 2019. *JAMA Network Open.* 2020;3(3). doi:10.1001/jamanetworkopen.2020.3976.

[21] Li W, Frank E, Zhao Z, Chen L, Wang Z, Burmeister M, et al. Mental health of young physicians in China during the novel coronavirus disease 2019 outbreak. *JAMA Network Open.* 2020;3(6):e2010705. doi:10.1001/jamanetworkopen.2020.10705.

[22] Schecter A, Diaz F, Moise N, Anstev DE, Ye S, Agarwal S, et al. Psychological distress, coping behaviors, and preferences for support among New York healthcare workers during the COVID-19 pandemic. *Gen Hosp Psychiatry.* 2020. September–October;66:1–8.

[23] Btaquehais MD, Vargas-Caceres S, Gomez-Duran E, Nieva G, Valero S, Casas M, et al. The impact of the COVID-19 pandemic on the mental health of healthcare professionals. *QJM.* 2020;113:613–617.

[24] Johnson SU, Ebrahimi OV, Hoffart A. PTSD symptoms among health workers and public service providers during the COVID-19 outbreak. *PLoS ONE.* October 21, 2020. doi: 10.1371/journal.pone.0241032.

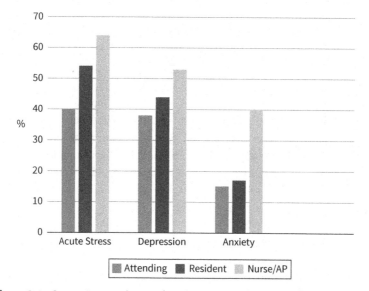

Figure 3.1. Stress, Depression, and Anxiety in Attendings, Residents, and Nurses.

From: Schecter A, Diaz F, Moise N, Anstev DE, Ye S, Agarwal S, et al. Psychological distress, coping behaviors, and preferences for support among New York healthcare workers during the COVID-19 pandemic. *Gen Hosp Psychiatry*. 2020 September–October;66:1–8.

pretty concerning decline in mood and increase in depressive symptoms. There's an increase in concern for patients, a feeling of not being able to do as much as they normally would. Then there's the added concern for themselves and their families. On one hand, they feel 'This is why I became a doctor.' On the other, it's 'I'm putting myself, my spouse, and my children at risk.' My sense is that stress and anxiety will be worse in places where clinicians feel that leadership is more concerned with finances than with safety, or is not being upfront about masks and P.P.E. Ultimately, you want to know that your institution is behind you."[25]

The suicide on April 26, 2020, of Dr. Lorna Breen, a New York City emergency medicine physician, made headlines in *The New York Times* and brought attention to the threat of suicide in HCWs during the pandemic.[26]

[25] Khullar D. The emotional evolution of coronavirus doctors and patients. *The New Yorker*. July 7, 2020.
[26] Knoll C, Watkins A, Rothfeld M. "I couldn't do anything": The virus and an E.R. doctor's suicide. *The New York Times*. July 11, 2020.

Breen had been working 12-hour shifts and supervising two different hospital emergency departments at the height of the pandemic. Her sister described her subsequent depression. "COVID broke her brain. She got crushed because she was trying to help other people. She got crushed by a nation that was not ready for this. We should have been prepared for this. We should have had some sort of plan."[27] Doctors commit suicide at twice the rate of the general population and 25% of ICU nurses have symptoms of PTSD.[28] Suicide ideation is present in 1 in 4 interns, 1 in 10 medical students, and 1 in 16 practicing physicians.[29] Dr. Chantal Brazeau, a psychiatrist at the Rutgers New Jersey Medical School, commented, "Physicians are often very self-reliant and may not easily ask for help. In this time of crisis, with high workload and many uncertainties, this trait can add to the load that they carry internally."[30] The increased stress that HCWs have faced during the pandemic has renewed efforts for greater focus on mental health treatment and suicide prevention in our profession.[31]

As beautifully summarized by Dzau and colleagues in the May 13, 2020, *New England Journal of Medicine*, "The inability to do their duty may be at the heart of the moral distress experienced by Covid-19 clinicians. With overwhelming numbers of seriously ill patients and shortages of essential supplies, providing the optimal standard of care becomes a mathematical impossibility. People who feel that they are called as healers in the altruistic Hippocratic tradition must stand by powerlessly as their patients sicken and die—a tragedy that can cause serious moral injury. Such injury may be most acute and long lasting in the young physicians, nurses, and other health professionals serving on the front lines during their formative years of training."[32]

[27] Wright L. The Plague Year. *The New Yorker*. December 28, 2020.

[28] Khullar D. The emotional evolution of coronavirus doctors and patients. *The New Yorker*. July 7, 2020.

[29] Menon NK, Shanafelt TD, Sinsky CA, Linzer M, Carlasare L, Brady KJS, et al. Association of physician burnout with suicidal ideation and medical errors. *JAMA Network Open*. December 9, 2020. 2020;3(12):e2028780. doi: 10.1001/jamanetworkopen.2020.28780.

[30] Hoffman J. "I can't turn my brain off": PTSD and burnout threaten medical workers. *The New York Times*. May 16, 2020.

[31] Leung TI, Angie Chen C-Y, Pendharkar S. Seeking and implementing evidence-based physician suicide prevention. *JAMA Intern Med*. June 29, 2020;180(9):1258. doi:10.1001/jamainternmed.2020.1841.

[32] Dzau VJ, Kirch D, Nasca T. Preventing a parallel pandemic-a national strategy to protect clinician's well-being. *N Engl J Med*. May 13, 2020. doi: 10.1056/NEJMp2011027.

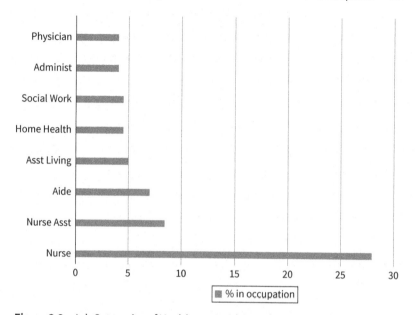

Figure 3.2. Job Categories of Healthcare Workers Infected with COVID-19.
From: CDC COVID Data Tracker. Accessed January 11, 2021.

As of January 11, 2021, there had been 350,000 cases of COVID-19 and 1,223 deaths in HCWs with nurses and nursing assistants making up the largest categories of hospitalized HCWs (Figure 3.2).[33] Frontline HCWs had a threefold greater risk for COVID infection compared to the general population.[34] In the United States the number of HCWs infected with COVID increased tenfold from April to December.[35] The median age in HCWs was 41 years and 79% were female. As in the general population, fatalities in HCWs were more prevalent in Asian and Black patients and those with chronic medical conditions.

[33] CDC COVID Data Tracker. Accessed January 11, 2021.
[34] Hughes MM, Groenewold MR, Lessem SE, Xu K, Ussery EN, Wiegand RE, et al. Update: Characteristics of health care personnel with COVID-19—United States, February 12–July 16, 2020. *MMWR*. September 25, 2020. 2020;69(38):1364–1368.
[35] Nguyen LH, Drew DA, Graham MS, Joshi AD, Guo C-G, Ma W, et al. Risk of COVID-19 among front-line healthcare workers and the general community: A prospective cohort study. *Lancet Public Health*. September 2020;5(9):e475–e483. doi: 10.1016/S2468-2667(20)30164-X.

In Los Angeles County, from the start of the pandemic to May 31, 10% of the 57,000 COVID cases were in HCWs.[36] Almost half were HCWs in long-term care facilities, 28% were working in hospitals, and 7% in medical offices. Nurses represented 50% of cases. About 5% were hospitalized, with 40 (0.7%) deaths. Work-related risk factors for COVID infections in HCWs have included working in a high-risk department, a diagnosed family member, inadequate hand hygiene, improper PPE use, close contact with patients (≥12 times/day), long daily contact hours (≥15 h), and unprotected exposure.[37] In six states, from March 1 to May 31, 2020, 6% of adults hospitalized with COVID-19 were HCWs.[38] The median age was 49 years, and 72% were female and 52% were Black. Ninety percent had at least one underlying medical disorder, and obesity was the most common comorbidity, present in 73%. Twenty-eight percent of the HCWs were admitted to an ICU, 16% required mechanical ventilation, and 4% died.

Paul Cary, a 66-year old retired paramedic and firefighter from Colorado, died from COVID on May 1, 2020. He was one of the thousands of HCWs who traveled to New York to help out at the peak of the pandemic. He had already signed up for a second 30-day deployment in New York when he began to feel ill. New York Mayor Bill de Blasio paid tribute to Cary: "We have lost someone who came to our aid, to our defense, and there's something particularly painful when someone does the right thing—a fellow American comes from across the country to try to help the people of New York City, and while working to save lives here, gives his own life. It's very painful."[39]

Even before the pandemic, some reports suggested that 50% of US physicians were experiencing professional burnout,[40] and the cost of physician burnout in the United States was estimated at $4.6 billion yearly, or $7,600

[36] Hartmann S, Rubin Z, Sato H, OYong K, Terashita D, Balter S. Coronavirus 2019 (COVID-19) infections among healthcare workers, Los Angeles County, February–May 2020. *Clin Infect Dis.* 2020 Aug 17;ciaa1200. doi: 10.1093/cid/ciaa1200.

[37] Shaukat N, Mansoor Ali D, Razzak J. Physical and mental health impacts of COVID-19 on healthcare workers: A scoping review. *Int J Emerg Med.* July 20, 2020;13(1):40. doi: 10.1186/s12245-020-00299-5.

[38] Kambhampati AK, O'Halloran AC, Whitaker M, Magill SS, Chea N, Chai SJ, et al. COVID-19-associated hospitalizations among health care personnel-COVID-NET, 13 states, March 1–May 31, 2020. *MMWR.* October 30, 2020;69(43):1576.

[39] Gross J. Colorado paramedic who came to help New York dies from Covid-19. *The New York Times.* May 2, 2020.

[40] Shanafelt TD, Noseworthy JH. Nine organizational strategies to promote engagement and reduce burnout. *Mayo Clin Proc.* November 18, 2016. doi.org/10.1016/j.mayocp.2016.10.004

per employed physician each year.[41] Early in the pandemic, more than one-half of HCWs from 60 countries had symptoms consistent with burnout.[42] Factors associated with increased stress and burnout in nurses from the United Kingdom included exhaustion, moral distress, difficulties communicating with masks, and being perceived as a threat to the safety of their general community.[43] Tammy Kocherhans, an ICU nurse in Utah, said, "These patients are different than the typical patient. They're very complex. They can change in the blink of an eye. And it's very hard as a nurse when you wrap your heart and soul into taking care of these patients. I started noticing that I was emotionally tired. I was physically completely exhausted. And I was beginning to question whether or not I could continue forward being a nurse at all. I was past my physical capacity."[44]

Dr. Eileen Barrett, director of graduate medical education at the University of New Mexico, said, "We came into this time with really unprecedented levels of burnout in the profession. It's always awful to have our health systems and our personal strengths tested. But in a time when people were feeling so much more stress, distress, and burnout in the profession, then it's particularly hard to have another layer on top of that. A lot of people have been experiencing professional loneliness and isolation having to do with spending more time behind screens, having less time with our patients, having less time with our peers."[45]

As the pandemic surged in the fall and winter of 2020, HCWs and hospitals found themselves in the same desperate situation as in March and April. The U.S. Strategic National Stockpile had only 115 million masks, far short of the recommended 300 million. Dr. Shikha Gupta, executive director of Get Us PPE, warned, "Health care workers are exhausted and frustrated, and it's really hard to believe that on Nov. 10, it feels very much like

[41] Han S, Shanafelt TD, Sinsky CA, Awad KM, Dyrbye LN, Fiscus LC, et al. Estimating the attributable cost of physician burnout in the United States. *Ann Intern Med.* June 4, 2019. doi: 10.7326/M18-1422.

[42] Morgantini LA, Naha U, Wang H, Francavilla S, Acar O, Flores JM, et al. Factors contributing to healthcare professional burnout during the COVID-19 pandemic. *PLoS One.* 2020;15(9):e0238217. doi: 10.1371/journal.pone.0238217.

[43] Maben J, Bridges J. Covid-19: Supporting nurses' psychological and mental health. *J Clin Nurs.* 2020;29:2742–2750. doi: 10.1111/jocn.15307.

[44] Becker A. What seven ICU nurses want you to know about the battle against covid-19. *The Washington Post.* December 7, 2020.

[45] Abbasi J. Prioritizing physician mental health as COVID-19 marches on. *JAMA.* May 20, 2020. 2020;323(22):2235–2236. doi: 10.1001/jama.2020.5205.

the middle of March all over again. We're hitting the highest numbers of caseload that we've ever seen, and we're running into the same problems that we've been having since Day 1."[46]

Deborah Burger, president of the largest organization of registered nurses, said on November 11, 2020, "We're 11 months into the pandemic, and the administration is still not adequately addressing the safety of health care workers and the safety of our communities. I've been a nurse for over 45 years, and I have never seen anything like this. It's like we're in 'The Twilight Zone.'"[47] HCWs behind the scenes, such as laboratory scientists and technicians, were also affected, as Chelsa Ashley, a medical laboratory scientist in Indiana, said, "There's that panicked feeling that I should have stayed to take care of our community samples. There's guilt, when you walk away. It's devastating. We're working as hard as we can."[48] Gary Solesbee, working with COVID-patients in Albuquerque, New Mexico, saw no sign of things letting up in December. "It feels like it's picking up, actually. We're bracing for a surge on top of a surge during the holidays. You get very fatigued. Patients are incredibly sick. You're on your feet all day, going in and out of rooms, putting on, taking off P.P.E. When I get home, I take my scrubs off and collapse. It's like nothing I've experienced before."[49] In early December 2020, Shalon Matthews, an emergency room nurse in New York, worried, "We need staff, we need help, we need resources. I'm fearful for my patients and I'm fearful that the same thing that happened back in March, it's going to happen again—and once again, we're not prepared."[50]

Drs. Wendy Dean and Simon Talbot expressed their frustration as the COVID cases swelled in Boston: "There is an epidemic in this country of not listening to those in distress. For months, health care workers have been trying to put out the fire of this pandemic bucket by bucket. They have been waiting for the public to realize the enormity of the threat and to accept the necessity of simple sacrifices for the greater good: wearing a mask, physical

[46] Stolberg SG, Weiland N, LaFraniere S, Jacobs A. The surging coronavirus finds a federal leadership vacuum. *The New York Times*. November 11, 2020.

[47] Stolberg SG, Weiland N, LaFraniere S, Jacobs A. The surging coronavirus finds a federal leadership vacuum. *The New York Times*. November 11, 2020.

[48] Wu KJ. "Nobody sees us": Testing-lab workers strain under demand. *The New York Times*. December 3, 2020.

[49] Khullar D. America is running out of nurses. *The New Yorker*. December 15, 2020.

[50] Closson T. Nurses are anxious and angry in 2nd wave: "We're not prepared." *The New York Times*. December 17, 2020.

distancing, and avoiding large gatherings. They have been waiting for elected leaders to call the country together and ask them to rise above their individual interests. They have been waiting for *someone* to see the enormous and growing risk that health care workers face."[51]

As the COVID vaccine arrived in December, Dr. Valerie Briones-Pryor, an internist, expressed renewed hope but it was short-lived. "I was one of the first people to get vaccinated in Kentucky. The whole thing was surreal. I walked onstage and pulled up my sleeve with the cameras rolling. A few people clapped when the needle went in. Some of us were crying. It felt like this amazing victory celebration, and then I went back to check on my patients. One coded on me that morning. Oxygen deprivation. He was my 27th covid death. But even with the vaccine, the reality in our hospital hasn't changed, and we've got months more to go. This pandemic has taken me through the stages of grief. There was that initial denial, and some people got stuck there. Then it was anger, and I definitely had that. I was mad at my neighbors because they were having people over. Then I was bargaining— maybe if we lock down or do this or that, it won't be so bad. Then depression. Then acceptance. It's great to know I'll have protection against this virus, but it's more than that. It's a profound relief. I can finally see a way out of this, even if we aren't there yet. It's a reason to hope."[52]

Hospitals

Every hospital in the United States was transformed overnight by the pandemic. In March 2020, hundreds of critically ill COVID patients in New York City were transferred to Bellevue Hospital. Postoperative recovery units and inpatient floors became ICUs. As Dr. Ofri described, "On Monday, March 23rd . . . the number of coronavirus patients admitted to Bellevue has tripled—there are now close to a hundred. The coronavirus has now taken over the entire I.C.U. It's as if all the other calamities—heart attacks, strokes, traumas, appendicitis—have evanesced on cue. Walking through the E.R. that evening, I notice that every patient is hooked up to a different

[51] Dean W, Talbot SG. Beyond burnout: For health care workers, this surge of Covid-19 is bringing burnover. *STAT*. November 25, 2020.

[52] Saslow E. I needed something good to happen. *The Washington Post*. December 19, 2020.

model of ventilator, each with its own arrangement of buttons, dials, and touchscreens."[53]

At the peak of the pandemic in every large city, hospitals were pushed to their limits, none more so than Elmhurst Hospital Center in the borough of Queens in New York City.[54] Elmhurst was forced to transfer non-COVID patients to other hospitals and was woefully short on ventilators. One of their doctors said, "The emergency room began filling up, with more than 200 people at times. Every chair in the waiting room was usually taken. Patients came in faster than the hospital could add beds; earlier this week, 60 coronavirus patients had been admitted but were still in the emergency room. One man waited almost 60 hours for a bed last week."[55] Mary T. Bassett, who led the New York City Department of Health and Mental Hygiene, pointed to the lack of resources at poorly funded hospitals like Elmhurst: "It's hard to look at the data and come to any other conclusion. We've known for a long time that these institutions are under-resourced. The answer should be to give them more resources."[56] Dr. Carol Horowitz, director of the Institute for Health Equity Research at Mount Sinai, noted, "Certain hospitals are located in the heart of a pandemic that hit on top of an epidemic of poverty and stress and pollution and segregation and racism."[57]

Most hospitals that serve minority communities are publicly funded, with their patients covered by Medicare, Medicaid, or uninsured. These hospitals have fewer resources and often lower clinical quality measures than hospitals with large private insurer patient populations. For example, in Los Angeles, hospitals with clinical quality above the national norm had allocated 23% of inpatient days to Medicaid patients compared with 54% of inpatient days for hospitals in the bottom two clinical quality categories.[58] Private insurers pay 200%–300% of Medicare rates to hospitals for the same level of care.

[53] Ofri D. The public has been forgiving. But hospitals got some things wrong. *The New York Times*. May 22, 2020. Accessed May 22, 2020. https://www.newyorktimes.com/
[54] Rothfeld M, Sengupta S, Goldstein J, Rosenthal BM. 13 deaths in a day: An "apocalyptic" coronavirus surge at an N.Y.C. hospital. *The New York Times*. March 25, 2020.
[55] Rothfeld M, Sengupta S, Goldstein J, Rosenthal BM. 13 deaths in a day: An "apocalyptic" coronavirus surge at an N.Y.C. hospital. *The New York Times*. March 25, 2020.
[56] Rosenthal BM, Goldstein J, Otterman S, Fink S. Why surviving the virus might come down to which hospital admits you. *The New York Times*. July 31, 2020.
[57] Rosenthal BM, Goldstein J, Otterman S, Fink S. Why surviving the virus might come down to which hospital admits you. *The New York Times*. July 31, 2020.
[58] Kaplan A, O'Neill D. Hospital price discrimination is deepening racial health inequity. *N Engl J Med*. December 21, 2020. https://catalyst.nejm.org/doi/full/10.1056/CAT.20.0593

A hospital treating a privately insured patient will receive three or four times the price for identical service as a publicly funded hospital in the United States or as any hospital in the United Kingdom. The added burden during the pandemic on poorly funded hospitals was felt throughout the United States.

Collaboration between hospitals was essential during each pandemic surge. In Boston, Dr. Paul Biddinger recounted the allocation of space and resources during the pandemic. "We agreed together who had capacity and how we should best try and urge transfers to be shared among hospitals, so that we would evenly balance the load and make sure there were ICU beds available. It helps skip a couple of steps or skip a couple of phone calls if you already knew at the outset that hospital X that day was not going to be able to provide that service."[59]

Integrated hospital systems were best suited to respond to the pandemic. Affiliated hospitals in New York City coordinated their response to the COVID pandemic, sharing the care of more than 5,000 hospitalized patients from March 10 to May 1, 2020.[60] Neurosurgical, cardiac and surgical ICUs, post-anesthesia units, and operating rooms were converted to COVID-19 ICUs. Northwell Health redeployed ambulatory staff to inpatient care teams constructed to ensure adequate expertise, learning, and protected time. Sleep apnea BiPAP machines were converted into ventilators. Hospital at home care, with extensive use of telemedicine, were employed in New York, Boston, and other metro areas. Medical students were utilized in innovative roles during the pandemic, such as in a family-centered care program in a North Carolina hospital ICU.[61] This was especially important to facilitate communication between family members and ICU teams with restricted ICU visitation during the pandemic. In Colorado, between March and July 2020, seven health systems partnered to care for 6,300 patients, accounting

[59] Kowalczyk L. After the surge: Hospitals prep to bring back regular patients while virus cases linger. *The Boston Globe*. May 2, 2020.

[60] Schaye VE, Reich JA, Bosworth BP, Stern DT, Volpicelli F, Shapiro NM, et al. Collaborating across private, community, and federal hospital systems: Lessons learned from the Covid-19 pandemic response in NYC. *N Engl J Med*. November–December 2020. doi: 10.1056/CAT.20.0343.

[61] Parks Taylor S, Short RT, Asher AM, Muthukkumar R, Sanka P. Family engagement navigators: A novel program to facilitate family-centered care in the intensive care unit during Covid-19. *N Engl J Med*. September 15, 2020. https://catalyst.nejm.org/doi/full/10.1056/cat.20.0396

for 98% of COVID-hospitalized patients in the state.[62] Facilitation of rapid patient transfers between hospitals and sharing of equipment and faculty allowed allocation of resources to areas that needed them the most.

Patients recovering from COVID infections often required prolonged, complex hospital care. A 30-bed, multidisciplinary COVID-19 recovery unit was established at New York-Presbyterian/Weill Cornell Medical Center, to best care for patients transitioning from the ICU to their next level of care.[63] Staff from neurology, hospital medicine, pulmonary medicine, nephrology, physical medicine and rehabilitation, psychiatry and nursing, social work, psychology, nutrition, and care coordination made up the team. The unit focused on individualized physical rehabilitation, communication, and socialization.

Post-discharge care for severely ill COVID patients was also a major challenge. Almost 1,400 COVID-19 patients were discharged from the New York Presbyterian Hospital system during a single week, and 30% required facility-level care.[64] A post-acute-care team, made up of social workers, physicians, and skilled nursing facility (SNF) administrators, met every morning to plan discharge options. Post-acute bed capacity was greatly expanded with 100 beds in five new COVID-19 SNFs. In addition to SNFs, COVID patients were discharged to acute rehabilitation and long-term acute care hospitals. The hospital partnered with various community services to provide temporary living accommodations, such as at local hotels, when home care was not available. When patients were discharged home, each patient was contacted within a day using a standardized protocol. Northwell Health in New York set up staff care coordinators and navigators for rapid and safe transition of COVID-19 patients back to their community.[65] Discharged patients were enrolled in a 2-week day care transition program structured on

[62] Valin JP, Gulley S, Keidan B, Perkins K, Savor Price C, Neff W, et al. Physician executives guide a successful Covid-19 response in Colorado. *N Engl J Med*. October 15, 2020. https://catalyst.nejm.org/doi/full/10.1056/CAT.20.0402

[63] Gupta R, Gupta A, Ghosh AK, Stein J, Lindsay L, Beckley A, et al. A paradigm for the pandemic: A Covid-19 recovery unit. *N Engl J Med*. May 29, 2020. https://catalyst.nejm.org/doi/full/10.1056/cat.20.0238

[64] Shapiro A, O'Toole N, Tinling-Solages D, McGarvey T, Tretola M, Dunphey P. Re-envisioning discharge planning and expanding post-acute care capacity during a pandemic. *N Engl J Med*. June 8, 2020. https://catalyst.nejm.org/doi/full/10.1056/CAT.20.0216

[65] Brown Z, Messaoudi C, Flynn A, Bleau H, Leska E, Khalilullah M, et al. Prompt launch of a rapid transitions care model prevents re-hospitalizations of Covid-19 patients. *N Engl J Med*. December 3, 2020. https://catalyst.nejm.org/doi/full/10.1056/CAT.20.0506

clinical, behavioral, and social parameters. Patients who received this service were 30% less likely to be rehospitalized within 14 days.

Many healthcare systems developed unique community COVID-19 management, preventing needless inpatient care. Cambridge Health Alliance, a community teaching public health system in Massachusetts, developed an outpatient respiratory clinic that reached out to primary care high-risk individuals with any potential COVID symptoms.[66] Physicians, nurses, and case managers triaged patients by phone or in-person and were able to care for the vast majority without emergency department or hospital admission. During the first month they evaluated 7,500 patients, most by telemedicine and 15% with a respiratory clinic visit. Community and hospital connections during COVID-19 identified neighborhood hotspots and fostered targeted communication to improve contact tracing and treatment.[67] The 50 community health workers at New York–Presbyterian Hospital and the NYU Grossman School of Medicine in the early months of the pandemic enrolled 3,400 people in patient portals and performed 9,600 wellness checks over the phone.[68]

The ability to transfer the sickest patients sometimes met resistance. Dr. Theodore Iwashyna, a professor of internal medicine at the University of Michigan, warned in October 2020, "As hospitals in much of the country face a surge in patients with Covid-19 and the threat of influenza this fall and winter, we must be on guard against attempts to restrict patient admissions or limit intensive-care capacity."[69] Some large hospitals in California refused to accept COVID-19 patients or delayed their transfer from smaller hospitals.[70] Dr. Paul Casey, chief medical officer at Rush University Medical Center, said that public health officials should be able to direct patients to hospitals that have the capacity and expertise to treat critically ill COVID

[66] John J, Council L, Zallman L, Blau J. Developing an intensive community Covid-19 management strategy: Helping our patients access patient-centered care across a continuum of Covid-19 disease needs. *N Engl J Med.* May 27, 2020. https://catalyst.nejm.org/doi/full/10.1056/CAT.20.0181

[67] Kosel KC, Nash DB. Connected communities of care in times of crisis. *N Engl J Med.* August 24, 2020. https://catalyst.nejm.org/doi/full/10.1056/CAT.20.0361

[68] Peretz PJ, Islam N, Matiz LM. Community health workers and Covid-19-Addressing social determinants of health in times of crisis and beyond. *N Engl J Med.* 2020;383:e108. doi: 10.1056/NEJMp2022641

[69] Iwashyna TJ. Do hospitals value everyone? This winter, they have a chance to prove it. *The New York Times.* October 30, 2020.

[70] Evans M, Berzon A, Hernandez D. some California hospitals refused Covid-19 transfers for financial reasons, state emails show. *The Wall Street Journal.* October 19, 2020.

patients. "Our philosophy was, there's going to be patients out there like we saw in New York City that, if there's not a coordinated response . . . there's going to be patients unfortunately that suffer and patients that end up dying that may have otherwise been saved."[71]

US hospitals lost more than $300 billion during the pandemic.[72] This was related to a 20% decrease in inpatient volume, a 35% decrease in outpatient volume, and a dramatic fall in elective surgery. Overall healthcare use declined by 23% in March 2020 and 52% in April with large drops in preventive care, including colonoscopy, mammograms, HbA1c, vaccinations, and elective procedures, including MRIs and cataract and joint surgery.[73] In the United Kingdom, at least 28 million elective operations were delayed during the first 3 months of the pandemic.[74] Hospitals that treated high numbers of coronavirus patients were hit the hardest, not only losing lucrative elective surgery but also suffering heavy costs from long patient stays in intensive care units. At Houston Methodist Hospital, during early April, surgical volume decreased by 78% and imaging studies by 56%.[75] Dr. David Blumenthal, president of the Commonwealth Fund, a health research organization, said, "Health care has always been viewed as recession-proof, but it's not pandemic-proof. The level of economic impact, plus the fear of coronavirus, will have a more dramatic impact than any event we've seen in the health care system in my lifetime."[76]

How to best restart hospital inpatient and ambulatory care as the pandemic persisted was a huge dilemma. At New York-Presbyterian, a Restart Coordination Committee focused on what consumers and providers will

[71] Schorsch K. During the pandemic, Chicago hospitals are on their own to transfer patients. *WBEZ Chicago.* June 29, 2020.

[72] American Hospital Association. New AHA report: Losses deepen for hospitals and health systems. June 30. 2020. https://www.aha.org/press-releases/2020-06-30-new-aha-report-losses-deepen-hospitals-health-systems

[73] Whaley CM, Pera MF, Cantor J, Chang J, Velasco J, Hagg HK, et al. Changes in health services use among commercially insured US populations during the COVID-19 pandemic. *JAMA Network Open.* November 5, 1020. 2020;3(11):e2024984. doi: 10.1001/jamanetworkopen.2020.24984.

[74] COVIDSurg Collaborative. Elective surgery cancellations due to the COVID-19 pandemic: Global predictive modelling to inform surgical recovery plans. *Br J Surg.* 2020;10.1002/bjs.11746.

[75] Tittle S, Braxton C, Schwartz RL, Siebenaler C, Sukin D, Boom ML, et al. A guide for surgical and procedural recovery after the first surge of Covid-19. *N Engl J Med.* July 2, 2020. https://catalyst.nejm.org/doi/full/10.1056/cat.20.0287

[76] Kliff S. Hospitals knew how to make money. Then Coronavirus happened. *The New York Times.* May 15, 2020.

demand of hospitals and how hospitals can provide a sense of confidence with reopening.[77] Key restarting items included centralized pre-procedure scheduling and testing. More urgent appointments and procedures were prioritized. Dr. Alastair Bell, chief operating officer at Boston Medical Center, said, "We have all gone from predicting the peak to predicting when we will be able to do other work that has been deferred. In all scenarios, there will be COVID. We are going to be managing in a dual world for some period of time, even for a long time. Ann Prestipino, senior vice president and incident commander at Massachusetts General Hospital, worried about patients who had waited for their procedures: "They are becoming urgent or emergency cases that we have to start doing . . . we have to start moving on them now."[78]

More than 1,300 patients at Vanderbilt University Medical Center were surveyed to discover what measures would need to be established to bring them back for their routine healthcare.[79] One-half were most anxious about catching COVID-19, especially from other patients. Only 40% expressed no hesitancy in going for their normal healthcare, although 80% said they would seek care immediately for an urgent problem. The majority wished to wait at least 1 month before any elective procedures and 10% planned on waiting more than 6 months.

Ramping elective procedures and surgery back up was based on urgency and safety. All patients needed to be tested for COVID-19 prior to any procedure or surgery, and various pathways to assure 100% compliance were utilized.[80] Timely testing and adequate PPE were essential. Total procedure time and turnaround time were increased due to COVID safety precautions. Large medical centers, in order to maintain at least 15% of beds for COVID-19 patients, kept their surgical volume at 70%–80% of baseline.[81] In the United Kingdom, it was predicted that until COVID-19 hospitalizations

---

[77] Forese LL, Corwin SJ. Restarting with Covid-19: Seven key action items. *N Engl J Med*. May 7, 2020. https://catalyst.nejm.org/doi/full/10.1056/CAT.20.0207

[78] Kowalczyk L. After the surge: Hospitals prep to bring back regular patients while virus cases linger. *The Boston Globe*. May 2, 2020.

[79] Patel S, Lorenzi N, Smith T, Carlson BR, Sternberg P. Critical insights from patients during the Covid-19 pandemic. *N Engl J Med*. July 13, 2020. https://catalyst.nejm.org/doi/full/10.1056/CAT.20.0299

[80] Hamilton BCS, Kratz JR, Sosa JA, Wick EC. Developing perioperative Covid-19 testing protocols to restore surgical services. *N Engl J Med*. June 19, 2020. https://catalyst.nejm.org/doi/full/10.1056/CAT.20.0265

[81] Tittle S, Braxton C, Schwartz RL, Siebenaler C, Sukin D, Boom ML, et al. A guide for surgical and procedural recovery after the first surge of Covid-19. *N Engl J Med*. July 2, 2020. https://catalyst.nejm.org/doi/full/10.1056/cat.20.0287

dropped to low levels, pre-pandemic volume of elective surgery would not be possible without use of field hospitals, private hospitals, and deployment of former and newly qualified staff.[82] Multidisciplinary reviews were essential to provide guidance on performing surgery and frequently subject to change.[83] Nonacute elective surgery scheduling should take into account the rate of new COVID-19 cases per 100,000 people as a 7-day average in the local community.[84] A study from the COVIDSurg Collaborative recommended that any person with a positive SARS-CoV-2 nasal swab test should have surgery delayed at least 1 month.[85]

The risk of nosocomial infection for hospitalized COVID-19 patients has been low, at 0%–2%.[86] At the University of Chicago Medical Center, restarting surgery was guided by the rubric Medically Necessary, Time-Sensitive System (MENTS), asking procedural questions, such as how long the surgery will take, how many physicians are needed, the degree of danger by waiting and predicting the risk of infection. As explained by Dr. Vivek Prachand, "This is meant to reassure patients, clinicians, and hospital leaders that the choices we're making have some basis other than our gut feelings. It's really a microcosm of what we need to do to open the economy. If we do it in a way that makes sense to people, that's transparent, that's dynamically adjustable, the public can feel confident that we know what we're doing."[87]

As of November 18, with the fall uptick in COVID infections, more than 1,000 US hospitals were critically short on staff.[88] Nasia Safdar, the medical director of infection control at the University of Wisconsin's hospital system, said, "I think capacity, in terms of staffing, is probably the biggest challenge

[82] McCabe R, Schmit N, Christen P, D'Aeth JC, Lochen A, Rizmie D, et al. Adapting hospital capacity to meet changing demands during the COVID-19 pandemic. *BMC Med.* October 16 2020;18(1):329. doi: 10.1186/s12916-020-01781-w.

[83] Tzeng C-WD, Tran Cao HS, Roland CL, Teshome M, Bednarski BK, Ikoma N, et al. Surgical decision-making and prioritization for cancer patients at the onset of the COVID-19 pandemic: A multidisciplinary approach. *Surg Oncol* September 2020. 2020;34:182–185. doi: 10.1016/j.suronc.2020.04.029.

[84] Wu K, Smith CR, Lembecke BT, Ferreira TBD. Elective surgery during the Covid-19 pandemic. *N Engl J Med.* 2020;383:1787–1790. doi: 10.1056/NEJMclde2028735.

[85] COVIDSurg Collaborative. Delaying surgery for patients with a previous SARS-CoV-2 infection. *Br J Surg.* 2020 Nov;107(12):e601–e602. doi:10.1002/bjs.12050.

[86] Wu K, Smith CR, Lembecke BT, Ferreira TBD. Elective surgery during the Covid-19 pandemic. *N Engl J Med.* 2020;383:1787–1790. doi: 10.1056/NEJMclde2028735.

[87] Khullar D. The coronavirus pandemic's wider health-care crisis. *The New Yorker.* June 29, 2020.

[88] McMinn S, Simmons-Duffin S. 1,000 U.S. hospitals are "critically" short on staff-and more expect to be soon. NPR. November 20, 2020.

that hospitals are facing right now. As we're seeing rates of infections rise in the community, we're seeing infections in our employees as well. While it's relatively easy to have a new bed come from somewhere, you really can't bring in a fully trained healthcare worker without a lot of challenges."[89] By mid-December 2020, there were more than 110,000 patients hospitalized daily in the United States, twice as many as during the worst days of April. Half of the states were experiencing critical staff shortages. ICU capacity was exhausted and ICU nurses, who normally care for two patients at a time, were often caring for eight at once.[90]

Once again, all elective procedures and surgery were canceled. Hospital floors became COVID units. Ambulances waited hours to offload critically ill patients into the hospital. Dr. Lewis Kaplan, head of the Society of Critical Care Medicine, said, "After having spent so many months dealing with all the pandemic-related things without a break, you're now asked to do it once more. That's part of our commitment as doctors, and yet a not-very-small part of you asks, 'Did it have to be this way?' And in your heart of hearts you're sure it really didn't."[91]

[89] McMinn S, Simmons-Duffin S. 1,000 U.S. hospitals are "critically" short on staff-and more expect to be soon. NPR. November 20, 2020. https://www.npr.org/sections/health-shots/2020/11/20/937152062/1-000-u-s-hospitals-are-short-on-staff-and-more-expect-to-be-soon

[90] Khullar D. America is running out of nurses. The New Yorker. December 15, 2020.

[91] Shammas B, Eunjung Cha A, Guarino B, Dupree J. Record numbers of covid-19 patients push hospitals and staffs to the limit. The Washington Post. December 16, 2020.

4

Impact on Primary Care and Specialty Care

Offices Shuttered

More than 1 million US healthcare jobs were lost during the first 6 months of the pandemic.[1] In April 2020, 90% of primary care physicians (PCPs) were not scheduling any routine healthcare visits, and 97% of all medical practices in the United States had experienced a loss of income related to COVID-19.[2] In-person visits fell by 65% in the United Kingdom from February to May 2020.[3]

. A survey of 400 PCP and specialty practices in Massachusetts between May 20 and July 9, 2020, reported a 44% reduction of in-person visits, as weighted by each full-time-equivalent (FTE) (Table 4.1).[4] PCP total revenues decreased by 54%. There was an increase in telehealth visits, but that made up for less than 50% of the lost revenue from inpatient visits.

About one-quarter of staff in these Massachusetts practices were furloughed or laid off during the pandemic. Sixty to eight percent of procedures, imaging, tests, and referrals were canceled or deferred, and there was a 24% net revenue reduction (Figure 4.1). Staff leaders said, "We are working twice as hard, for half the result. It is exhausting and disheartening.

[1] U.S. Department of Labor. Unemployment Insurance Weekly Claims. Washington: U.S. Department of Labor, July 20, 2020. Accessed August 19, 2020. https://www.dol.gov/ui/data.pdf.
[2] Lewis C, Seervai S, Shah T, Abrams MK, Zephyrin L. Primary care and the COVID-19 pandemic. The Commonwealth Fund. April 22, 2020. August 2020;70(697):e540–e547. https://doi.org/10.26099/73k0-a831.
[3] Joy M, McGagh D, Jones N, Liyanage H, Sherlock J, Parimalanathan V, et al. Reorganisation of primary care for older adults during COVID-19. Br J Gen Pract. July 13, 2020. August 2020;70(697):e540–e547. doi: 10.3399/bjgp20X710933.
[4] Song Z, Giuriato M, Lillehaugen T, Altman W, Horn DM, Barnett KG, et al. Economic and clinical impact of Covid-19 on provider practices in Massachusetts. N Engl J Med. September 11, 2020. https://catalyst.nejm.org/doi/full/10.1056/CAT.20.0441

Table 4.1 Changes in Monthly Visits, before and during Pandemic, 2020 (per FTE)

In-Person	In-Person	Telehealth	Telehealth
Before Pandemic	During Pandemic	Before Pandemic	During Pandemic
205	115	0	33

From: Song Z, Giuriato M, Lillehaugen T, Altman W, Horn D, Philips R, et al. Economic and clinical impact of Covid-19 on provider practices in Massachusetts. *N Engl J Med Catalyst.* September 11, 2020. https://catalyst.nejm.org/doi/full/10.1056/CAT.20.0441

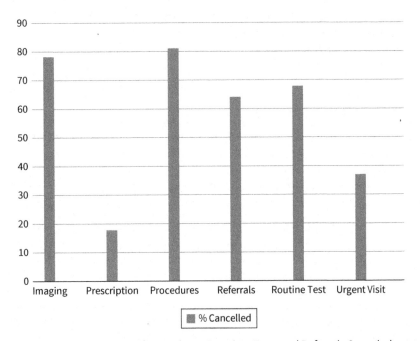

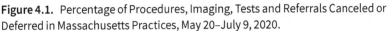

Figure 4.1. Percentage of Procedures, Imaging, Tests and Referrals Canceled or Deferred in Massachusetts Practices, May 20–July 9, 2020.

From: Song Z, Giuriato M, Lillehaugen T, Altman W, Horn DM, Barnett KG, et al. Economic and clinical impact of Covid-19 on provider practices in Massachusetts. *N Engl J Med.* September 11, 2020.

Everyone, providers and staff, is burning out. I have never until now feared for my practice's viability. I don't think any amount of financial assistance will get us to pre-Covid-19 operation levels."[5]

Toward the end of April 2020, three primary care organizations told Alex Azar, the Secretary of Health and Human Services, "The situation facing front-line physicians is dire. Obstetrician-gynecologists, pediatricians, and family physicians are facing dramatic financial challenges leading to substantial layoffs and even practice closures."[6]

A number of ongoing surveys of PCPs from across the United States detailed the progression of changes in practices during the pandemic. By mid-September, only 20% of PCPs were at pre-pandemic revenue levels despite one-quarter permanently reducing their staff size.[7] It was estimated that primary care practices lost $67,774 in gross revenue per FTE during 2020, a loss of $15 billion for the nation's PCPs.[8]

About 8% or 16,000 medical practices closed during the pandemic.[9] More than 15% of community health centers, providing care to 30 million Americans, had closed as of May 1, 2020.[10] Pediatricians, the lowest paid PCPs, were the most vulnerable. Dr. Susan Sirota, a pediatrician in Chicago said, "This virus has the potential to essentially put pediatricians out of business across the country. Our waiting rooms are like ghost towns."[11] Dr. Ryan Kearney, a pediatrician at Northampton Area Pediatrics in western Massachusetts, said, "What was a day typically spent seeing upwards of 30-plus kids became seeing anywhere from 8 to 15 children on telemedicine."[12]

[5] Song Z, Giuriato M, Lillehaugen T, Altman W, Horn DM, Barnett KG, et al Economic and clinical impact of Covid-19 on provider practices in Massachusetts. *N Engl J Med*. September 11, 2020. https://catalyst.nejm.org/doi/full/10.1056/CAT.20.0441

[6] Abelson R. Doctors without patients: "Our waiting rooms are like ghost towns." *The New York Times*. May 5, 2020.

[7] Primary Care Collaborative. Quick COVID-19 primary care survey. September 18–21, 2020. www.pcpcc.org.

[8] Basu S, Phillips RS, Phillips R, Paterson LE, Landon BE. Primary care practice finances in the United States amid the COVID-19 pandemic. *Health Affairs*. June 25, 2020;39;9. https://doi.org/10.1377/hlthaff.2020.00794.

[9] Abelson R. Doctors are calling it quits under stress of the pandemic. *The New York Times*. November 15, 2020.

[10] Kishore S, Hayden M. Community health centers and Covid-19-Time for congress to act. *N Engl J Med*. August 20, 2020. doi:10.1056/NEJMp2020576.

[11] Abelson R. Doctors without patients: "Our waiting rooms are like ghost towns." *The New York Times*. May 5, 2020.

[12] Horn D. The pandemic could put your doctor out of business. *The Washington Post*. April 24, 2020.

Dr. Kelly McGregory, a pediatrician in practice near Minneapolis, lamented, "As an independent practice with no real connection to a big health system, it was awful. I did some telemedicine, but it wasn't enough volume to really replace what I was doing in the clinic. It was devastating. That was my baby."[13]

It was estimated that 60,000 primary care practices would eventually close because of the pandemic.[14] Small and midsize independent PCP practices were hit the hardest financially. Currently 50% of US family medicine physicians are in practice with five or fewer healthcare providers and 50% of the 220,000 PCPs in the US work as full- or part-owners of independent small practices.[15] Michael Chernow, a health policy professor at Harvard Medical School, said, "I worry about how well these practices will be able to shoulder the financial burden to be able to meet the health care needs people have. If practices close down, you lose access to a point of care."[16]

During the past decade, many small PCPs have been bought up by hospitals and that process accelerated during the pandemic. Dr. Christopher Crow, a PCP in Texas, said, "The hospitals are getting massive bailouts. They've really left out primary care, really all the independent physicians. Here's the scary thing—as these practices start to break down and go bankrupt, we could have more consolidation among the health care systems."[17] Keeping PCPs open and functioning during the pandemic was crucial to preventing hospitals from becoming overwhelmed. At least one-third of ER visits can be avoided with a well-functioning PCP system, particularly when patients can access same-day appointments easily.[18]

Dr. Daniel Horn, a PCP at Massachusetts General Hospital, said, "I'm lucky to work for a well-funded, nonprofit hospital system, where expensive advanced testing and difficult procedures like bone marrow and heart transplants help subsidize the money-losing work my primary-care peers do to

---

[13] Abelson R. Doctors are calling it quits under stress of the pandemic. *The New York Times.* November 15, 2020.

[14] Horn D, Altman W, Song Z. Primary care is being devastated by Covid-19. It must be saved. *STAT.* April 29, 2020.

[15] Basu S, Phillips RS, Phillips R, Paterson LE, Landon BE. Primary care practice finances in the United States amid the COVID-19 pandemic. *Health Affairs.* June 25, 2020;39(9). https://doi.org/10.1377/hlthaff.2020.00794.

[16] Abelson R. Doctors are calling it quits under stress of the pandemic. *The New York Times.* November 15, 2020.

[17] Abelson R. Doctors are calling it quits under stress of the pandemic. *The New York Times.* November 15, 2020.

[18] Yoon J, Cordasco KM, Chow A, Rubenstein LV. The relationship between same-day access and continuity in primary care and emergency department visits. *PLoS One.* September 2, 2015. doi: 10.1371/journal.pone.0135274.

sustain the health of our communities. If it was a standalone business, a high functioning primary-care network like mine would operate at a net loss of 20 to 30% a year, or an average annual cost of $150,000 per physician . . . That's partly because we employ diabetes educators, geriatric case managers, social workers and addiction-recovery coaches—health professionals who are essential to the well-being of our patients but whose work is not reimbursed by insurers. But these are unsure times even at Mass General: We project a 50% loss in patient-care volume over 3 to 4 months, which will have a major impact on the $1.2 billion annual revenue our 2,900 physicians bring in. We hope that our infrastructure and assets will help us weather the storm. Most primary-care doctors in our country don't have this support system. America began this pandemic with a national primary-care shortage, and without help, they now face existential peril."[19]

Dr. Beverly Jordan, a family medicine physician in Enterprise, Alabama, was barely able to keep open during the pandemic, hanging on with the money paid out from the government's Paycheck Protection Program. "For the first time in my career, we're really just planning short-term. We've never had this level of insecurity."[20] PCPs were under enormous financial, emotional, and physical stress, as recounted by Cortney Barry, a family nurse practitioner in Soledad, California. "Like this is just such a high level of stress and just keeps going. The other hard part is there's no end in sight. My intention is to stay in medicine, although I would not be totally opposed to doing something in a totally different area, which is something that I would not have said in the past."[21]

Primary Care Soldiers On

The traditional office visit was dismantled during the pandemic. Primary care clinicians adapted, delivering care despite closed offices and a barebones staff. Telemedicine was critical to that. On May 1, 2020, at one large PCP, 93% of patient visits were by phone or video.[22] Digital thermometers and pulse

---

[19] Horn D. The pandemic could put your doctor out of business. *The Washington Post*. April 24, 2020.

[20] Marks C. America's looming primary-care crisis. *The New Yorker*. July 25, 2020.

[21] Abelson R. Doctors are calling it quits under stress of the pandemic. *The New York Times*. November 15, 2020.

[22] Myers G, Price G, Pykosz M. A report from the Covid front lines of value-based primary care. *N Engl J Med*. May 1, 2020. https://catalyst.nejm.org/doi/full/10.1056/CAT.20.0148

oximeters were sent to patients, a COVID-19 hot line was set up with daily virtual team rounds on all infected patients. More than 5,000 daily virtual wellness check-ups were done.

Early in the pandemic, video consultations in the United Kingdom went from 3% to 95% of all PCP visits.[23] Australia appropriated $1.1 billion in support of the COVID response in primary care, establishing a national call center and setting up general-practice-led respiratory centers.[24] The United Kingdom, which had already increased primary care funding during its NHS Five Year Forward View, added significant government funds to help the primary care crisis.[25] Still more than 10% of UK PCPs were at risk of closing because of fiscal pressure,[26] and 40% reported lack of adequate mental health support during the pandemic.[27]

Some in the United Kingdom saw a silver lining with the pandemic-enforced fewer face-to-face visits.[28] The United Kingdom's typical 10-minute appointments had been considered too short and their care continuity lower than in most countries with similar healthcare systems, such as Canada and Germany.[29] Rather than the typical 10-minute PCP appointments in the United Kingdom, visits during the pandemic were lengthened and made more personal, adhering to the Royal College of General Practitioner's decision to "re-invigorate relationship-based medicine."[30]

[23] Sharma SC, Sharma S, Thakker A, Roshan M, Varakantam V. Revolution in UK general practice due to COVID-19 pandemic: A cross-sectional survey. *Cureus.* 2(8):e9573. August 5, 2020. doi: 10.7759/cureus.9573.

[24] Desborough J, Dykgraaf SH, de Toca L, Davis S, Roberts L, Kelaher C, et al. Australia's national COVID-19 primary care response. *Med J Aust.* July 4, 2020. 213(3):104–106.e1. doi: 10.5694/mja2.50693.

[25] Sharma SC, Sharma S, Thakker A, Roshan M, Varakantam V. Revolution in UK general practice due to COVID-19 pandemic: A cross-sectional survey. *Cureus.* 2;8:e9573. August 5, 2020. doi: 10.7759/cureus.9573.

[26] Sharma SC, Sharma S, Thakker A, Roshan M, Varakantam V. Revolution in UK general practice due to COVID-19 pandemic: A cross-sectional survey. *Cureus.* 2;8:e9573. August 5, 2020. doi: 10.7759/cureus.9573.

[27] Trivedi N, Trivedi V, Moorthy A, Trivedi H. Recovery, restoration and risk: A cross sectional survey of the impact of COVID-19 on general practitioners in the first UK city to lockdown. *Br J Gen Pract Open.* November 16, 2020. 2020;BJGPO.2020.0151. doi: 10.3399/BJGPO.2020.0151.

[28] Gray DP, Freeman G, Johns C, Roland M. Covid 19: A fork in the road for general practice. *BMJ.* September 28, 2020. doi: 10.1136/bmj.m3709.

[29] Tzortziou V, Gregory S, Pereira Gray D. The power of personal care: The value of the patient-GP consultation. *Br J Gen Pract.* 2020:70:596597. doi: https://doi.org/10.3399/bjgp20X713717.

[30] Royal College of General Practitioners. Policy and campaigning priorities 2020. https//www.rcgp.org.uk

Many practices set aside specific space and time for the evaluation of patients with potential COVID infection. Large family medicine practices, including at the Mayo Clinic, converted practices to COVID care clinics, integrating triage, respiratory, and continuing care.[31] Many pediatricians scheduled well-child visits exclusively in the morning and sick visits in the afternoon. Dr. Yul Ejnes, a primary care physician in Rhode Island, redesigned his office waiting room. "The waiting room was a problem even before covid-19. You'd have twenty-five people sitting next to each other. Some of them were there for a flu shot, others were there with the flu—throw in coronavirus and that setting is totally unacceptable."[32]

Community-wide testing and patient education were coordinated among PCPs and medical centers. A mobile free testing program developed at the University of North Carolina (UNC Health) tested 2,000 patients for COVID-19 in 2 months, including 70% minority patients and 63% uninsured.[33] Testing was combined with patient education, free PPE, and scheduled follow-up care. Community health sites, such as provided by the Dallas, Texas, Connected Community of Care Program, promoted COVID-19 education. "We have seen first-hand that written/graphic communications delivered to community residents in-person through familiar food pantries, homeless shelters, and places of worship are effective in getting the message into the hands of a vulnerable population."[34]

The fallout from canceling inpatient visits and conversion to telemedicine increased many PCPs' concerns about loss of autonomy and personal connection. Dr. Paquita de Zuleta, a general practitioner in the United Kingdom, said, "Losing touch threatens to undermine our relationships with our patients, our professional practice, and a key element of our pedagogy. Clearly, we are still in the midst of the pandemic and difficult balancing acts are being made on a daily basis between avoiding potentially harmful, or even lethal, contagion and avoiding harm to social bonds and livelihoods (blandly called

---

[31] Jacobson NA, Nagaraju D, Miller JM, Bernard ME. COVID Care Clinic: A unique way for family medicine to care for the community during the SARS-CoV-2 (COVID-19) pandemic. *J Prim Care Community Health*. October 22, 2020. doi: 10.1177/2150132720957442.

[32] Khullar D. The coronavirus pandemic's wider health care crisis. *The New Yorker*. June 29, 2020.

[33] Towns R, Corbie-Smith G, Richmond A, Gwynne M, Fiscus L. Rapid deployment of a community-centered mobile Covid-19 testing unit to improve health equity. *N Engl J Med*. October 22, 2020.

[34] Kosel KC, Nash DB. Connected communities of care in times of crisis. *N Engl J Med*. August 24, 2020.

'the economy'). The physical examination should remain a 'touchstone' of general practice."[35] Dr. Paul Hyman, a PCP in Brunswick, Maine, agreed: "As our primary care practice has pivoted to telehealth and the physical examination has been ripped away from me, I find myself reflecting on what value the examination has. The physical examination remains a place where I offer something of distinct value that is appreciated. In the past 10 years, with the emergence of the electronic health records and team-based care, we primary care physicians have found ourselves on unsure footing with our identity and way of practicing frequently shifting and disrupted. But the pandemic has forced me to deconstruct my routine, including the physical examination, in a way that leaves me on uncertain ground. This has been emotionally exhausting and unsettling."[36]

Team primary care management was a major focus during the pandemic. Many states lifted burdensome restrictions on PCP utilization and supervision of nurse practitioners.[37] Chronic care home management and remote patient monitoring allowed PCPs to expand home care and to generate much needed revenue. These services often involved clinical care managers visiting patients' homes, senior centers, and long-term care facilities, supported virtually by PCPs.[38] Medical assistants were also given greater independence, often serving as the healthcare coach for patients and families.[39]

The pandemic fortified the connection of PCPs to their community. In the United Kingdom, PCPs worked closely with local councils and community groups to improve patient equity, as outlined in the Royal College of General Practice Health Inequalities Standing Group.[40] As part of the NHS's efforts to promote self-care, UK PCPs were provided regular access to a "link worker" implementing community social interactions, with a goal to reach 1 million

---

[35] De Zuleta P. Touch matters: COVID-19, physical examination, and 21st century general practice. *Br J Gen Pract.* 2020;70(701):594–595. doi: https://doi.org/10.3399/bjgp20X713705.

[36] Hyman P. The disappearance of the primary care physical examination-losing touch. *JAMA Intern Med.* 2020;180:1417–1418. doi: 10.1001/jamainternmed.2020.3546.

[37] Bluth R. California resists push to lift limits on nurse practitioners during Covid-19 pandemic. *STAT.* April 17, 2020.

[38] Donohue D. A primary care answer to a pandemic: Keeping a population of patients safe at home through chronic care management and remote patient monitoring. *Am J Lifestyle Med.* June 29, 2020. 2020;14(6):595–601. doi: 10.1177/1559827620935382.

[39] Chapman SA, Blash LK. New roles for medical assistants in innovative primary care practices. *Health Serv Res.* 2017;52:383–406. doi: 10.1111/1475-6773.12602.

[40] Ashwell G, Blane D, Lunan C, Matheson J. General practice post-COVID-19: Time to put equity at the heart of health systems. *Brit J Gen Pract.* 2020;70:400. doi: https://doi.org/10.3399/bjgp20X712001

patients by 2024.[41] Specific targets included exercise and weight loss intervention, community activities, and self-help groups.

In the United States, the Health Resources and Services Administration (HRSA) supports 1,400 community health centers providing primary care to 30 million primarily underserved patients.[42] HRSA administered weekly COVID-19 surveys to track testing and patient data, categorized by race/ ethnicity. The CDC and HRSA jointly evaluated survey data for the weeks of June 5–October 2, 2020, which included test results of more than 3 million individuals, of which 36% were Hispanic and 20% Black.

By October 1, 2020, ambulatory visits in many US PCP practices were returning to pre-pandemic levels.[43] However, PCPs were still having difficulty accessing essential supplies. In the fall of 2020, 20% of PCPs were struggling to find PPE and COVID tests.[44] The US government had spent more than $200 billion to shore up the healthcare system, but little of that was earmarked for primary care. Andy Slavitt, a former administrator for Medicare and Medicaid, noted, "The typical primary care doctor received only enough to keep his or her practice open for one week. We need to target assistance directly to small independent physician practices. They should not be competing with multibillion-dollar health systems and other businesses for the same funds."[45] As doctors were the first in line to get vaccinated for COVID-19, once again PCPs were last in that line. As of December 15, 2020, less than one-quarter of the United States' PCPs had been scheduled to receive a vaccine.[46] Dr. Jason Lofton, a PCP in Arkansas, said, "We feel like we're the true front line. We see these patients before they go to the hospital or ER. We want to make sure we're not forgotten. It's easy when you're in a small corner of

[41] Roland M, Everington S, Marshall M. Social prescribing—Transforming the relationship between physicians and their patients. *N Engl J Med*. July 9, 2020. doi: 10.1056/NEJMp1917060.

[42] Romero L, Pao LS, Clark H, Riley C, Merali S, Park M, et al. Health center testing for SARS-ScV-2 during the COVID-19 pandemic-United States, June 5–October 2, 2020. *MMWR*. 2020;69;50:1895–1901. doi: 10.15585/mmwr.mm6950a3.

[43] Mehrotra A, Chernew M, Linetsky D, Hatch H, Cutler D, Schneider EC. The impact of the COVID-19 pandemic on outpatient care: Visits return to prepandemic levels, but not for all providers and patients. *The Commonwealth Fund*. October 15, 2020. https://doi.org/10.26099/41xy-9m57

[44] Primary Care Collaborative. Quick Covid-19 Primary Care Survey. September 18–21, 2020.

[45] Slavitt A, Mostashari F. Covid-19 is battering physician practices. They need help now. *STAT*. May 28, 2020.

[46] Goldhill O, "Still waiting for my turn": Primary care doctors are being left behind in the vaccine rollout. *STAT*. January 4, 2021.

rural America to be left out."[47] The 220,000 US PCPs provide over half of the approximately 1 billion office visits annually in the United States, including 85% of the care for the most common chronic health issues, such as hypertension and diabetes.[48] About 50% of our PCPs operate within the community in independent small practices.

Dr. Horn and colleagues suggested that the United States provide "financial relief to primary care practices by switching from fee for service to a monthly bundled payment . . . provide all primary care practices nationwide with a reasonable fixed payment, say on average $50 per patient per month. This fixed payment would replace any previous fee-for-service payments the practice would have received during this time. Practices that serve patients with greater health needs could receive a larger budget than those that serve healthier patients, a risk-adjustment process used by most public and private payers today. Envision the following: You go to your primary care practice amid a bout of depression and are immediately able to see a behavioral health provider. You struggle with alcohol use or opioid addiction and a recovery coach checks in with you weekly as you pursue recovery. Your loved one develops dementia and a nurse case manager helps coordinate his or her care. If we change the way we pay for primary care, that's the kind of care our nation could attain."[49]

Specialty Care

Cardiologists and neurologists were directly involved in the care of hospitalized COVID-19 patients, and their ever-expanding role has been discussed throughout this book. However, the daily activities and practice of every medical and surgical specialist was impacted by the pandemic.

For the most part, oncology care was able to continue during the pandemic, facilitated by a rapid and near-total switch to telemedicine for the most vulnerable patients. Infusion sites were consolidated and refigured to

[47] Goldhill O, "Still waiting for my turn": Primary care doctors are being left behind in the vaccine rollout. *STAT*. January 4, 2021.

[48] Basu S, Phillips RS, Phillips R, Peterson LE, Landon BE. Primary care practice finances in the United States amid the COVID-19 pandemic. *Health Affairs*. June 25, 2020. https://doi.org/10.1377/hlthaff.2020.00794.

[49] Horn D, Altman W, Song Z. Primary care is being devastated by Covid-19. It must be saved. *STAT*. April 29, 2020.

minimize exposure. Many infusions were moved to a patient's home, such as Penn Medicine's Cancer Care at-home program, which, over 7 weeks, increased home infusions from 39 to 310 patients.[50] Continuing these oncology telemedicine and home programs will require that insurers provide appropriate long-term telemedicine reimbursement.

In a UK national cancer registry of 1,044 confirmed COVID-19 cases between March 18 and May 8, 2020, hematologic malignancies were associated with increased hospitalizations, but leukemia was the only cancer conclusively linked to an increase in COVID-related death.[51] Professor Rachel Kerr, Senior Researcher at the University of Oxford, said, "Using these new data, we are working fast to identify trends and correlations, which will enable us to create a tiered risk assessment tool so we can more precisely define the risk to a given cancer patient and move away from a blanket 'vulnerable' policy for all cancer patients."[52]

Obstetrics met a number of challenges with COVID-19. Pregnancy increases the risk of severe COVID-19 infection, with a threefold greater risk of pregnant women requiring ICU and mechanical ventilation and a 70% increased mortality risk compared to nonpregnant women.[53] Risk factors for poor outcome for pregnant women with COVID mirrored those in the general population, including obesity and minority status. One of the study authors, Dr. Sascha Ellington, noted, "We are now saying pregnant women are at increased risk for severe illness. Previously we said they 'might be' at increased risk for severe illness. The absolute risk of these severe outcomes is low among women 15 to 44, regardless of pregnancy status. Pregnant women should be counseled about the importance of seeking prompt medical care if they have symptoms."[54] Preterm births have been more common in women

---

[50] Laughlin AI, Begley M, Delaney T, Zinck L, Schuchter LM, Doyle J, et al. Accelerating the delivery of cancer care at home during the Covid-19 pandemic. *N Engl J Med.* July 7, 2020. https://catalyst.nejm.org/doi/full/10.1056/cat.20.0258

[51] Lee LYW, Cazier J -B, Starkey T, Briggs SEW, Arnold R, Bisht V, et al. COVID-19 prevalence and mortality in patients with cancer and the effect of primary tumor subtype and patient demographics: A prospective cohort study. *Lancet Oncol.* 2020;21:1309–1316. doi: 10.1016/S1470-2045(20)30442-3.

[52] Blood cancer patients are most vulnerable to COVID-19. Oxford University Research. August 25, 2020.

[53] Zambrano LD, Ellington S, Strid P, Galang RR, Oduyebo T, Tong VT, et al. Update: Characteristics of symptomatic women of reproductive age with laboratory-confirmed SARS-CoV-2 infection by pregnancy status-United States, January 22–October 3, 2020. *MMWR.* November 2, 2020. 2020;69(44):1641–1647.

[54] Rabin RC. Pregnant women face increased risks from Covid-19. *The New York Times.* November 2, 2020.

who tested positive for the virus. There has been conflicting evidence regarding an increased rate of stillbirths and neonatal deaths during the pandemic.[55,56] Increases in stillbirths in the general population may have been related to the hesitancy to seek medical care. Every pregnant woman should be tested for COVID-19, but, as Dr. Laura Jelliffe-Pawloski noted, this results in more anxiety. "Women are expressing so much fear about being infected, but also about going to the hospital, delivering and being separated from their child."[57]

Preexisting chronic illness increased the risk for COVID-related morbidity and mortality, necessitating careful attention to disease management. This was well documented in patients with diabetes, who had a threefold greater mortality risk. For patients with type 1 and type 2 diabetes, optimal blood glucose monitoring and management were essential but became very challenging, because of social isolation, lack of exercise, and dietary restrictions, especially problematic in poorer communities.

During the pandemic, there was an increase in diabetic ketoacidosis in children and adolescents with newly diagnosed diabetes and more cases of severe ketoacidosis and hyperosmolarity requiring very high doses of insulin in patients with preexisting diabetes.[58,59] The increased risk of unusual insulin requirements and the potential need to readjust or change other hypoglycemic medications during COVID-19 infections required close consultation with endocrinologists. Metformin was associated with decreased mortality in women with obesity or type 2 diabetes who were hospitalized with COVID-19.[60] The protective mechanism is not well understood. A randomized, controlled trial of dapagliflozin, a sodium-glucose cotransporter

[55] Khalil A, von Dadelszen P, Draycott T, Ugwumadu A, O'Brien P, Magee L. Change in the incidence of stillbirth and preterm delivery during the COVID-19 pandemic. *JAMA*. 2020;324:705–706. doi:10.1001/jama.2020.12746.

[56] Handley SC, Mullin AM, Elovitz MA, Gerson K, Montoya-Williams, D, Lorch SA, et al. Changes in preterm birth phenotypes and stillbirth at 2 Philadelphia hospitals during the SARS-CoV-2 pandemic, March–June 2020. *JAMA*. 2021;325(1):87–89. doi: 10.1001/jama.2020.20991.

[57] Gammon K. The psychic toll of a pandemic pregnancy. *The New York Times*. December 14, 2020.

[58] Kamrath C, Monkemoller K, Biester T, Roher TR, Warncke K, Hammersen J, et al. Ketoacidosis in children and adolescents with newly diagnosed type 1 diabetes during the COVID-19 pandemic in Germany. *JAMA*. July 20, 2020;324(8):801–804.

[59] Rubino F, Zimmet P, Alberti G, Bornstein S, Eckel RH, Mingrove G, et al. New-onset diabetes in Covid-19. *N Engl J Med*. June 12, 2020. 383:789–790. doi: 10.1056/NEJMc2018688.

[60] Bramante CT, Ingraham NE, Murray TA, Marmor S, Hovertsen S, Gronski J, et al. Metformin and risk of mortality in patients hospitalized with COVID-19: A retrospective cohort analysis. *The Lancet*. December 3, 2020. https://doi.org/10.1016/S2666-7568(20)30033-7

inhibitor, which has renal and cardiac protective benefits in patients with type 2 diabetes, will determine whether it may decrease COVID-19 morbidity and mortality in high-risk patients.[61]

I am most familiar with the impact of the pandemic on my own field of rheumatology, but there are some similar, general observations across all medical subspecialties:

- There is no convincing evidence that the pandemic has increased the incidence of immune/inflammatory diseases, such as rheumatoid arthritis, inflammatory bowel disease, psoriasis, or multiple sclerosis.
- There have been reports of unique inflammatory/immune disorders associated with COVID-19 infections, such as the multisystem inflammatory disorder, vasculitic/purpuric skin lesions, a reactive arthritis, and various neurologic and gastrointestinal syndromes. These have been rare and generally self-limited and likely immune mediated.
- Each subspecialty has established a set of guidelines for use of immunosuppressive medications during the pandemic, with explicit instructions for hospitalized patients.
- Comorbid disease severity correlates closely with COVID-related morbidity and mortality, so optimal management of the underlying disease is essential.
- Subspecialties have set up national and international registries to track the outcome of their patients during and after COVID-19 infections and more observations will be forthcoming in the near future.

Primary care providers and specialists were forced to innovate and cut back on waste during the pandemic. These lessons learned will promote value-based care in the future.

Kosiborod M, Berwanger O, Koch GG, Martinez F, Mukhtar O, Verma S, et al. Effects of dapagliflozin on prevention of major clinical events and recovery in patients with respiratory failure due to COVID-19. *Diabetes Obes Metab.* December 15, 2020. 2021 Apr;23(4):886–896. doi:10.1111/dom.14296.

5
Telemedicine

Office Practice

The COVID-19 pandemic pushed telemedicine to the center of medical services. Early in the pandemic, hospitals and physician practices were exclusively using telephone visits to field all COVID-related questions, to coordinate testing, and to triage clinical care.[1] During the first quarter of 2020, the number of telehealth visits skyrocketed in the United States, notably after March 6, 2020, when the Centers for Medicare & Medicaid Services loosened regulations and improved payments for telemedicine.[2] This allowed physicians to be paid the same amount for telephone and video visits as for in-person visits. The removal of geographic boundaries and widening of eligible platforms, like Zoom or FaceTime, allowed greater accessibility for patients and providers. In January and February 2020, telehealth patient encounters for possible COVID-19 infection at four centers in the United States averaged 5,000–7,000 visits weekly, but in early March they averaged 15,000–20,000 visits weekly.[3]

In March 2020, the United Kingdom announced the essential role of virtual care during the pandemic. "The NHS will take a digital-first approach to accessing primary care and outpatient appointments in an attempt to reduce the total footfall into practices, protecting both staff and patients."[4]

[1] Mehrotra A, Ray K, Brockmeyer DM, Barnett ML, Bender JA. Rapidly converting to "virtual practices": Outpatient care in the era of Covid-19. *N Engl J Med*. April 1, 2020. https://catalyst.nejm.org/doi/full/10.1056/CAT.20.0091

[2] Koonin LM, Hoots B, Tsang CA, Leroy Z, Farris K, Jolly B, et al. Trends in the use of telehealth during the emergence of the COVID-19 pandemic—United States, January–March 2020. *MMWR*. October 30, 2020. 2020;69;43:1595–1599. doi: 10.15585/mmwr.mm6943a3.

[3] Koonin LM, Hoots B, Tsang CA, Leroy Z, Farris K, Jolly B, et al. Trends in the use of telehealth during the emergence of the COVID-19 pandemic—United States, January–March 2020. *MMWR*. October 30, 2020. 2020;69;43:1595–1599. doi: 10.15585/mmwr.mm6943a3.

[4] Joy M, McGagh D, Jones N, Liyanage H, Sherlock J, Parimalanathan V, et al. Reorganisation of primary care for older adults during COVID-19. *Br J Gen Pract*. July 13, 2020. 2020;70(697):e540–e547. doi: 10.3399/bjgp20X710933.

Shortly thereafter, 80%–90% of PCP visits in the United Kingdom were virtual. Dr. Sam Wessely, a London general practitioner, said, "We're basically witnessing 10 years of change in one week. It used to be that 95 percent of patient contact was face-to-face: You go to see your doctor, as it has been for decades, centuries. But that has changed completely."[5] Dr. Paul Deffley, a general practitioner in Southern England, talked about the importance of virtual visits for his nursing home patients. "The risk I pose to residents of a nursing home by going in there is pretty significant, yet they are some of our most frail patients. Being able to eyeball someone, to engage in a consultation with them and assess for clinical signs, is an absolute game changer for how we're able to safely manage people."[6]

In the United Kingdom, a COVID-19 consultation guideline provided instructions for video set-up recommended techniques for obtaining a virtual history and examination.[7] These UK investigators later developed a remote assessment tool for patients who would need escalation to a higher level of care.[8] UK PCPs accepted the rapid switch to virtual care but noted that more patient/provider input was important in moving ahead with telemedicine. "Remote patient consultations (phone, message, video) have become the norm across all care settings and accepted by patients—this needs to continue. Digital innovation has been escalated and blockers have been removed to accelerate transformational change . . . inadequate training, education and even limited trust are hurdles we must overcome. We can see that there needs to be a much greater focus on helping staff and patients gain the skills to make the most of the switch to digital. There needs to be a continued drive towards a digitally-enabled, holistic health service where the patient is truly part of the team and the decision-making process."[9]

[5] Mueller B. Telemedicine arrives in the U.K.: "10 years of change in one week." *The New York Times*. April 5, 2020.

[6] Mueller B. Telemedicine arrives in the U.K.: "10 years of change in one week." *The New York Times*. April 5, 2020.

[7] Greenhalgh T, Koh GCH, Car J. Covid-19: A remote assessment in primary care. *BMJ*. 2020;368. doi: 10.1136/bmj.m1182.

[8] Greenhalgh T, Thompson P, Weiringa S, Neves AL, Husain L, Dunlop M, et al. What items should be included in an early warning score for remote assessment of suspected COVID-19? *BMJ Open*. November 12, 2020. doi: 10.1136/bmjopen-2020-042626.

[9] Royal Society of Medicine. Survey results: Comprehensive insights into how COVID-19 has impacted healthcare. RSM. https://blog.hettshow.co.uk/healthtech-state-of-play-round-up-infographic. Accessed October 1, 2020.

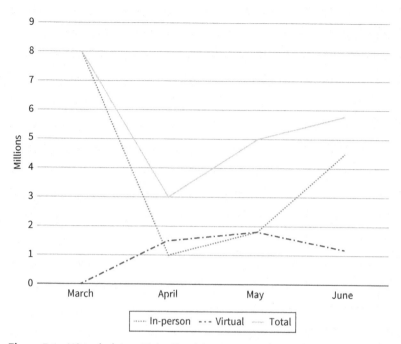

Figure 5.1. US Ambulatory Visits, Total, In-Person and Virtual, March–June 2020.

Modified from: Fox B, Sizemore JO. Telehealth: Fad or the future. Epic Health Research Network. August 18, 2020.

PCPs in the United States were slower to fully adopt telemedicine and even by late March 2020, 60% of PCP offices were not doing any telehealth visits.[10] There was a sharp decline in all US ambulatory visits in late March accompanied by a gradual increase in telehealth visits over the next 3 months (Figure 5.1).[11] By August, more than 70% of PCPs were using telemedicine, 50% said they planned to increase its use, and 12% had switched to a primarily telemedicine practice.[12] One-third of the telehealth visits were only by telephone since many patients lacked access to video technology or

[10] Primary Care Collaborative. Primary Care & COVID-19: Week 2 Survey. Primary Care Collaborative; March 26, 2020. https://www.pcpcc.org/2020/03/26/primary-care-covid-.

[11] Fox B, Sizemore JO. Telehealth: Fad or the future. Epic Health Research Network. August 18, 2020. info@ehrn.org

[12] The Physicians Foundation. 2020 Physician Survey. Part 1. August 18, 2020. Physiciansfoundation.org

Table 5.1 Weekly In-Person vs. Virtual Visits/1,000 Medicare Insurance Members

Week	February 1–6	April 1–7	May 1–7	June 1–7
In-Person Visits/1,000	125	58	40	64
Virtual Visits/1,000	0.8	10	31	24

From: Patel SY, Mehrotra A, Huskamp HA, Uscher-Pines L, Ganguli I, Barnett ML. *JAMA Int Med.* November 16, 2020. Trends in outpatient care delivery and telemedicine during the COVID-19 pandemic in the US.

were not comfortable with its use.[13] Among a national sample of 17 million Americans with Medicare Advantage insurance, between January and June 2020, there was a 2000% increase in telemedicine visits and a 30% decrease in in-person visits.[14] That decrease in in-person visits and increase in telemedicine visits was most notable from April 1 to June 1, 2020 (Table 5.1).

In less than 1 week, Central Ohio Primary Care provided telehealth services at their 70 practice sites to more than 350 physicians.[15] In PCP practices in Massachusetts, there were no telehealth visits before March 2020, but after March 2020, there were an average of 51 telehealth visits monthly for each provider.[16] Ezekiel Emanuel and Amol Navathe, who direct the Healthcare Transformation Institute at the University of Pennsylvania, noted: "Telemedicine is now everywhere. For years doctors resisted telemedicine, either because it was too hard to learn or, worse, because they made more money from an in-office visit. Last year just 22% of family physicians surveyed used video visits, according to the American Academy of Family Physicians. This is crucial because telemedicine is cost-efficient for matters that do not need physical contact and easier to work into patients' daily life, and it frees up office visits for patients with complex conditions. It

[13] Jaklevic MC. Telephone visits surge during the pandemic, but will they last? *JAMA.* 2020;324(16):1593–1595. October 7, 2020.
[14] Patel SY, Mehrotra A, Huskamp HA, Uscher-Pines L, Ganguli I, Barnett ML. Trends in outpatient care delivery and telemedicine during the COVID-19 pandemic in the US. *JAMA Int Med.* November 16, 2020. 2021;181(3):388–391.
[15] Stone RL. How an Ohio-based physician organization overcame internal hurdles and launched a telehealth service as Covid-19 shutdowns loomed. *N Engl J Med.* October 8, 2020.
[16] Song Z, Giuriato M, Lillehaugen T, Altman W, Horn DM, Barnett KG, et al. Economic and clinical impact of Covid-19 on provider practices in Massachusetts. *N Engl J Med. Catalyst.* Catalyst.nejm.org. September 11, 2020.

also makes it easier for doctors to provide after-hours care, reducing costly emergency room and urgent care clinic visits."[17]

Initially, many patients bemoaned the loss of in-person visits. One of Dr. Amy Wheeler's patients told her secretary, "Tell the doctor I have no interest in a phone call or one of those video visits. When she is back to seeing patients again in the office, let me know."[18] Over time, more and more patients expressed enthusiasm for telemedicine. Jane Brody, *New York Times* medical columnist wrote, "Even if no other good for health care emerges from the coronavirus crisis, one development—the incorporation of telemedicine into routine medical care—promises to be transformative. Using technology that already exists and devices that most people have in their homes, medical practice over the internet can result in faster diagnoses and treatments, increase the efficiency of care, and reduce patient stress."[19] Ninety-five percent of patients from a large primary care practice in New York City were satisfied with video visits during the COVID pandemic and 50% preferred virtual compared to in-person visits.[20] Ninety percent of Medicare Advantage beneficiaries had a positive experience with telehealth during the pandemic and 80% intended to use it for their future healthcare.[21]

Trueman Mills, an 86-year-old patient with congestive heart failure, valued his first virtual visit and not having to make the 90-mile trip to see his cardiologist in Pittsburgh. "I was very impressed by the whole operation. If we get out of this, we might find that a lot more medicine gets done this way, for good or for bad."[22] Avoiding travel and long waits in offices and the overall cost savings were most often prized by patients. Not infrequently, patients admitted that they felt more comfortable discussing personal problems virtually. Dr. Robert Bart, chief medical information officer at the University of Pittsburgh Medical Center, observed, "One of the comments

[17] Emanuel EJ, Navathe AS. Will 2020 be the year that medicine was saved? *New York Times*. April 14, 2020.

[18] Wheeler AE, My patients want the good old days of office visits. That's not happening any time soon. *STAT*. July 22, 2020.

[19] Brody JE. A pandemic benefit: The expansion of telemedicine. *The New York Times*. May 12, 2020.

[20] Sinha S, Kern LM, Gingras LF, Reshetnyak E, Tung J, Pelzman F, et al. Implementation of video visits during COVID-19: Lessons learned from a primary care practice in New York City. *Front Public Health*. September 17, 2020. doi: 10.3389/fpubh.2020.00514.

[21] Minow NH, Boucher R. Congress should make sure telemedicine is here to stay. *The Boston Globe*. July 16, 2020.

[22] Ross C. In fading steel towns, chronically ill patients hope video visits stay after the pandemic goes. *STAT*. April 29, 2020.

we most frequently get from patients is that they have more face time with the physician during these telemedicine visits than they do when they're in person. The satisfaction rate among patients is remarkably high."[23] Bart helped design the university's Rapid Access Video Evaluation to ensure that patients got connected to the correct specialist and to determine whether virtual care was reasonable. "We want to work with our specialists and primary care physicians along disease states to figure out how care should be delivered for patients who have diabetes or lupus."[24]

A consensus of suggestions to best prepare practices for telemedicine and to optimally engage patients included the following:[25,26,27,28]

- Practice with technology, including camera set-up and connectivity and upgrade technology if needed. Use of two monitors, one for video consultation and one for the electronic health records. When possible, a staff member, such as medical assistant, should be the designated telemedicine navigator. Prepare the patient for video guidance well ahead of initial appointments.
- Providers should practice listening techniques and use open-ended questions, like "you scheduled this visit because . . ." Focus on the patient and be present. Use a quiet, private place. Offer patients and family a "virtual waiting room."
- Verbalize clearly when referring to the electronic medical record (EMR) since the patient likely cannot see it.
- Recognize that COVID-19-related stress and anxiety may affect patients' attentiveness. Look for emotional cues. Involve family members.
- Present information in small portions. Provide a short summary of the visit. Ask patients if there are any remaining questions.

[23] Ross C. In fading steel towns, chronically ill patients hope video visits stay after the pandemic goes. *STAT*. April 29, 2020.

[24] Ross C. Telehealth grew wildly popular amid COVID-19. *STAT*. September 1, 2020.

[25] Millstein JH, Kindt S. Reimagining the patient experience during the Covid-19 pandemic. *N Engl J Med*. June 24, 2020. https://catalyst.nejm.org/doi/full/10.1056/CAT.20.0349

[26] Cooley L. Fostering human connection in the Covid-19 virtual health care realm. *N Engl J Med*. May 20, 2020. https://catalyst.nejm.org/doi/full/10.1056/CAT.20.0166

[27] Car J, Choon-Huat Koh G, Foong PS, Wang CJ. Video consultations in primary and specialist care during the covid-19 pandemic and beyond. *BMJ*. October 20, 2020;371. doi: 10.1136/bmj.m3945.

[28] Hrountas S, Bier AJ, Green S. A post Covid new normal: Developing fundamental changes for group medical practices. *N Engl J Med*. November 25, 2020. https://catalyst.nejm.org/doi/full/10.1056/CAT.20.0427

A virtual physical examination often required added video assistance from the patient or family, such as moving the camera to best show a rash or a swollen leg. Home measures of blood pressure, oxygen saturation, temperature, and body weight can be taken and recorded before the visit.[29]

It immediately became apparent that a large swath of the general population was not ready or able to participate in telemedicine without specific guidance and training. It was estimated that 30%–40% of older adults in the United States would be unable to use video visits because of technology issues and another 20% would have difficulty with telephone visits, primarily related to hearing or cognitive issues.[30]

Large Healthcare Organizations and Hospitals

Hospitals and affiliated healthcare centers adopted telemedicine almost overnight. Duke Health was averaging 100 video visits per month in 2019, but by April 2020 they were doing 2,000 virtual visits daily, and Partners Healthcare in Boston went from 0.8% to >70% of virtual visits in 6 weeks.[31] At Kaiser Permanente, virtual care visits went from 38% in February to a peak of 87% in April but were still at 77% in July 2020.[32] Their financial setback from the decrease of in-person visits was largely offset by a doubling of virtual care visits. E-visits for COVID-19 increased rapidly and by March 15 accounted for 56% of the total of 46,000 e-visits.

In just a few weeks, virtual visits at Stanford Health Care in California skyrocketed from 2% to more than 70%.[33] What was envisioned as a 2-year gradual telemedicine rollout happened in less than 1 month. More than 20,000 virtual health visits, including 15,000 video visits, were conducted in the first 2 months of the program. In a single day they performed 3,000

[29] Car J, Choon-Huat Koh G, Foong PS, Wang CJ. Video consultations in primary and specialist care during the covid-19 pandemic and beyond. *BMJ*. 2020;371:m3945. doi: 10.1136/bmj.m3945.

[30] Lam K, Lu AD, Shi Y, Covinsky KE. Assessing telemedicine unreadiness among older adults in the United States during the COVID-19 pandemic. *JAMA Int Med*. 2020;180(10):1389–1391. August 3, 2020.

[31] Haas L, Sharp C. Five takeaways digital health system leaders learned through Covid-19 response efforts. *N Engl J Med*. November 20, 2020.Catalyst.nejm.org.

[32] Robinson J, Borgo L, Fennell K, Funahashi TT. The Covid-19 pandemic accelerates the transition to virtual care. *N Engl J Med*. September 10, 2020. Catalyst.nejm.org

[33] Srinivasan M, Phadke AJ, Zulman D, Israni ST, Madill ES, Savage TR, et al. Enhancing patient engagement during virtual care: A conceptual model and rapid implementation at

ambulatory video visits, a fifty-fold increase over its baseline rate. The Stanford Virtual Health Care Clinical Process Model assigned virtual care responsibilities to the patient, to clinical and education teams, and to medical assistants for specific activities[34]:

- Patient responsibilities
  o Visit readiness
  o Watch health-related videos
  o Perform self-examination
  o Engage with primary health provider
- Medical assistant and digital health team responsibilities
  o Technology access, support, home metrics
  o Vitals, health screening
  o Digital lending library
- Patient and medical assistant
  o Agenda setting
  o Implement care plan
  o Health maintenance plan

Chris Van Gorder, President and CEO, described the rollout of telemedicine at Scripps Health in California: "In the face of this pandemic, we condensed a planned 18-month rollout of our telemedicine program to just 9 days. We went from zero telemedicine visits in October, to a handful of doctors being trained and us all being very excited when the first video visit was conducted in November, to where we are now: some 2,000 telehealth visits a day, conducted by more than 800 providers across primary care and specialty care lines including oncology, cardiology, neurology, and endocrinology. Through our telemedicine program, patients can use our Symptom Checker to assess their symptoms and get next steps on how to get appropriate care. E-visits are another option, and work by patients submitting a

an academic medical center. *N Engl J Med*. July 10, 2020. https://catalyst.nejm.org/doi/full/10.1056/CAT.20.0262

[34] Srinivasan M, Phadke AJ, Zulman D, Israni ST, Madill ES, Savage TR, et al. Enhancing patient engagement during virtual care: A conceptual model and rapid implementation at an academic medical center. *N Engl J Med*. July 10, 2020. https://catalyst.nejm.org/doi/full/10.1056/CAT.20.0262

brief questionnaire for diagnosis and treatment from a Scripps provider in 30 minutes. And finally, video visits allow patients to talk with one of our providers now or schedule a visit for another time. This change has been well received by our patients and clinicians, and it is a change that will be here to stay after this pandemic is over."[35]

Remote monitoring of COVID-19-infected patients at the University of Pennsylvania Health System was done with the aid of a "COVID Watch" that generated twice daily check-ins.[36] Text queries focused on respiratory symptoms and any patient self-reporting worse symptoms was contacted by a nurse within 1 hour. Over 3,000 patients enrolled in the program in the first month, and 83% of patients were managed by the automated program without in-person care. The Cleveland Clinic went from 10% to 70% virtual visits during the first few months of the pandemic with more than 80% of patients reporting that they were satisfied with the change.[37] They also designed a home-based telemedicine program for monitoring high-risk patients with COVID-19 infections and as of late May 2020 enrolled 2,000 patients in their team-based program.

Although the Veterans Administration (VA) health system was an early adopter of telehealth in the United States, the vast majority of outpatient care at VA hospitals and clinics was in-person until the pandemic. From March to the end of May 2020, the number of weekly video visits at VAs increased from 10,000 to 60,000 for mental healthcare, from 1,000 to 20,000 for primary care, and from 1,000 to 30,000 for specialty care and rehabilitation (Figure 5.2).[38] Telephone visits increased by 131%. E-consultation visits also increased, especially for diabetes and pulmonary medicine. Most patients were first-time users of telehealth, and many had little technology experience; those patients usually chose telephone rather than video conferencing. In the first 2 months of the pandemic, the VA loaned out more than 7,000

[35] NEJM Catalyst. Lessons from CEOs: Health care leaders nationwide respond to the Covid-19 crisis. *N Engl J Med*. July 29, 2020. https://catalyst.nejm.org/doi/full/10.1056/CAT.20.0150

[36] Morgan AU, Balachandran M, Do D, Lam D, Parambath A, Chaiyachati KH, et al. Remote monitoring of patients with Covid-19: Design, implementation, and outcomes of the first 3,000 patients in COVID watch. *N Engl J Med*. July 21, 2020. https://catalyst.nejm.org/doi/full/10.1056/CAT.20.0342

[37] Medina M, Babiuch C, Card M, Gavrilescu R, Zafirau W, Boose E, et al. Home monitoring for COVID-19. *Clev Cl J Med*. June 2020. doi: 10.3949/ccjm.87a.ccc028.

[38] Heyworth L, Kirsh S, Zulman D, Ferguson JM, Kizer KW. Expanding access through virtual care: The VA's early experience with Covid-10. *N Engl J Med*. July 1, 2020. Catalyst.nejm.org.

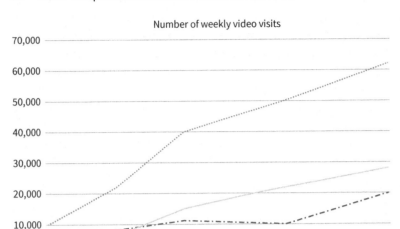

Figure 5.2. Increase in Virtual Healthcare Visits at US VA Hospitals, March–May 2020.

From: Heyworth L, Kirsh S, Zulman D, Ferguson JM, Kizer KW. Expanding access through virtual care: The VA's early experience with Covid-10. *N Engl J Med.* July 1, 2020.

tablets to patients. Critical to the success of telehealth in the VA system was the ability of staff to provide care across state lines.

Telemedicine visits should seamlessly interact with the EMR, and this is best integrated with patient portal accessibility. Before the pandemic, only about 30% of the general population were viewing their medical records online through patient portals.[39] Many large hospitals and health centers saved money and time by not integrating telemedicine into patient portals but rather relying on personal devices, smartphones, and tablets.

Telemedicine allowed collaboration from experts at distant medical centers during the pandemic. A critical care telemedicine program, with

---

[39] Haas L, Sharp C. Five takeaways digital health system leaders learned through Covid-19 response efforts. *N Engl J Med.* November 20, 2020. catalyst.nejm.

combined expertise from 20 clinicians at the University of Pittsburgh Medical Center and the Mayo Clinic, helped to manage COVID-19 patients in the ICU and the clinicians concluded: "It is possible to imagine future conditions that would facilitate the flexible deployment of telemedicine across states and systems to mitigate disparities in access to critical care expertise (for example, in rural or resource-limited hospitals), regardless of pandemic conditions."[40] High-intensity telemedicine costs more than $50,000–$100,000 annually per covered bed.

A weekly Zoom meeting of more than 200 critical care experts from around the world provided a "collaboration between centers that did not exist before. Now places in Texas, Florida, and Arizona are able to gain information from what the hospitals in the Northeast went through. That's the best thing coming out of these meetings and a silver lining for the Covid era."[41] The tele-ICU hub at Dartmouth-Hitchcock Medical Center connected its ICU physicians to clinicians caring for a critically ill patient at a small community hospital in New Hampshire. They were able to "Zoom in on Patient X, watch his cardiac monitor, and talk to the doctor, nurses, and paramedic on the scene. Electronic-record-sharing allowed them to 'chart on' the patient—to have real-time access to his vitals and his medications, just as though they were there."[42]

Penn Medicine created a web platform with comprehensive information and counseling opportunities described as "Created by patients, caregivers, staff, and providers, the Penn Medicine Listening Lab is a storytelling initiative that embraces the power of listening as a form of care."[43] Penn Medicine also designed a COVID-19 chatbot to provide accurate, updated information around the clock, serving an unlimited number of callers.[44] Boston Children's Hospital and Stanford Medicine developed population telehealth surveys, the National Daily Health Survey and the Covid Near You tool, to

---

[40] Barbash IJ, Sackrowitz RE, Gajic O, Dempsey TM, Bell S, Millerman K, et al. Rapidly deploying critical care telemedicine across state health systems during the Covid-19 pandemic. *N Engl J Med.* July 22, 2020. https://catalyst.nejm.org/doi/full/10.1056/CAT.20.0301

[41] Winslow R. How a Zoom forum is changing the way ICU doctors treat desperately ill Covid-19 patients. *STAT.* August 6, 2020.

[42] Seabrook J. The promise and the peril of virtual health care. *The New Yorker.* June 22, 2020.

[43] Millstein JH, Kindt S. Reimagining the patient experience during the covid-19 pandemic. *N Engl J Med.* June 24, 2020. https://catalyst.nejm.org/doi/full/10.1056/CAT.20.0349

[44] Herriman M, Meyer E, Rosin R, Lee V, Washington V, Volpp KG. Asked and answered: Building a chatbot to address Covid-19-related concerns. *N Engl J Med.* June 18, 2020. catalyst.nejm.org

predict prevalence and severity of infections in various parts of the country and provide health information.[45]

Mental Health and Specialty Care

Telepsychiatry had been used effectively before the pandemic, notably after prior natural disasters in the United States and the United Kingdom.[46] Mental health professionals quickly adopted to telemedicine during the pandemic with three-quarters of psychologists using only teletherapy in the later part of 2020.[47] Telemedicine visits for anxiety, depression, overactivity, bipolar disorder, insomnia, and opioid use disorder went from 3% of all visits before the pandemic to 66% during the second quarter of 2020.[48] Virtual mental health visits across the VA Health System increased sevenfold, from 7,500 to 52,600 in the first 2 months of the pandemic.[49] Research prior to the pandemic had previously shown that telehealth effectively expanded the access to mental health services and that virtual therapy was as effective as in-person therapy for the treatment of depression and posttraumatic stress disorder (PTSD).[50,51]

The psychiatry outpatient clinic at Houston Methodist Hospital had been transitioning to digital care prior to the pandemic and on March 18 switched to 100% telehealth care.[52] There was widespread acceptance of virtual

[45] Haas L, Sharp C. Five takeaways digital health system leaders learned through Covid-19 response efforts. *N Engl J Med.* November 20, 2020. catalyst.nejm.org.

[46] Torous J, Wykes T. Opportunities from the coronavirus disease 2019 pandemic for transforming psychiatric care with telehealth. *JAMA Psychiatry.* 2020;77:1205–1206. doi:10.1001/jamapsychiatry.2020.1640.

[47] American Psychological Association. Psychologists embrace telehealth to prevent the spread of COVID-19. APA Services Practice Resources. June 5, 2020.

[48] Mansour O, Tajanlangit M, Heyward J, Mojtabi R, Alexander GC. Telemedicine and office-based care for behavioral and psychiatric conditions during the COVID-19 pandemic in the United States. *Ann Intern Med.* November 17, 2020. doi: 10.7326/M20-6243.

[49] Carey B. The psychiatrist will see you online now. *The New York Times.* August 28, 2020.

[50] Acierno R, Gros D, Ruggiero KJ, Hernandez-Tejada BMA, Knapp RO, Lejuez CW, et al. Behavioral activation and therapeutic exposure for posttraumatic stress disorder: A noninferiority trial of treatment delivered in person versus home-based telehealth. *Depress Anxiety.* May 2016;33;5:415–423. doi:10.1002/da.22476.

[51] Ruskin PE, Silver-Aylaian M, Kling MA, Reed SA, Bradham DD, Hebel JR, et al. Treatment outcomes in depression: Comparison of remote treatment through telepsychiatry to in-person treatment. *Amer J Psych.* August 1, 2004. doi: 10.1176/appi.ajp.161.8.1471.

[52] Sasangohar F, Bradshaw MR, Carlson MM, Flack JN, Fowler JC, Freeland D, et al. Adapting an outpatient psychiatric clinic to telehealth during the COVID-19 pandemic: A practice perspective. *J Med Internet Res.* October 22, 2020. 2020;22(10):e22523. doi: 10.2196/22523.

therapy by patients and providers. Patient engagement in group therapy increased. Therapists expressed that there was value in being able to see patients in their home surroundings, especially for younger patients, providing "a much deeper level of knowing the child and understanding what their world might really be like. Being able to do the exposure in her room was so much more powerful."[53] Dr. Peter Yellowlees, who coauthored a textbook on telepsychiatry, shared this opinion: "From a clinical point of view, you can often learn more over video than in person, because you see people moving in their natural habitat, where they live, maybe how they interact with others. My office, by contrast, is not a neutral space. Your home is your space. It's more egalitarian, less stressful. And potentially you can turn the device off and end the session, if you really wanted."[54]

Most concerns about teletherapy were centered on protecting privacy as well as the aforementioned technology glitches. Lori Gottlieb, a psychotherapist, said, "My patients sheltering at home have had to find a place for their therapy sessions where nobody else can hear them. Sometimes they find privacy in a bedroom or a closet or a car, but often it's in a bathroom, with my patient sitting on a toilet seat while we speak."[55] Some therapists regretted the loss of visual and body language emotional cues, as expressed by Dr. Andres Sciolla, a psychiatrist at U.C. Davis: "In terms of trauma, one of the things many of us track is microexpressions, these flickers of emotional tone, when people are talking. I cannot tell you how many times I have noticed a flicker of tears or fear in the gaze of a patient, perceived a shift in feeling, and explored that—and found a lot behind that change."[56]

Initial reluctance to switch to teletherapy soon abated, as Dr. Tamara Greenberg, a psychologist in San Francisco, retold. "I thought it wasn't a *real* form of therapy, but I would say it's really been one of the most surprising, and in many ways pleasurable, experiences of my professional career."[57] Most patients also accepted the trade-offs of virtual versus in-person teletherapy, as Michael Raymos said, "There is a drop of social contact, not being able to

[53] Wilser J. Teletherapy, popular in the pandemic, may outlast it. *The New York Times.* July 9, 2020.

[54] Carey B. The psychiatrist will see you online now. *The New York Times.* August 28, 2020.

[55] Gottlieb L. In psychotherapy, the toilet has become the new couch. *The New York Times.* April 22, 2020.

[56] Carey B. The psychiatrist will see you online now. *The New York Times.* August 28, 2020.

[57] Wilser J. Teletherapy, popular in the pandemic, may outlast it. *The New York Times.* July 9, 2020.

always see his expression. There's more of an intimacy level when you're one on one and that office door is closed. But there's a comfort level at home. I'll sit there in bed with my dog, Bug, on my lap, and that comfort allows me to talk about things I maybe wouldn't have in the office, because of how painful they are. And I like not having to make that drive."[58]

Mental health integration of telemedicine will likely pave the way for its more widespread use throughout all of medicine. As stated by Shore and colleagues, "The development of telepsychiatry will likely be viewed in the future in terms of the eras before, during, and after COVID-19. The field of psychiatry, working with our colleagues in the wider field of medicine, has an opportunity now to proactively look at the current telemedicine regulations and begin advocating for their longer-term maintenance. This work could usher in a golden era for technology in psychiatry in which we are able to harmonize the benefits of telepsychiatry and virtual care while maintaining the core of our treatment: that of human connectedness."[59]

Most medical specialists pivoted to telemedicine quite seamlessly during the pandemic. Even in specialties that rely heavily on a physical examination, such as dermatology and orthopedics, telemedicine provided creative flexibility. Virtual visits were suitable for triaging and managing common dermatologic and musculoskeletal conditions, particularly as patients learned to readjust camera angles.

Gastroenterologists from 56 countries reported that during the pandemic more than 75% of their visits were by telemedicine, and they estimated that after the pandemic 25%–50% of visits would continue to be virtual.[60] Dr. Corey Siegel, a Dartmouth-Hitchcock gastroenterologist, noted, "I won't say anything good has come out of covid-19. But we've done almost seven hundred telemedicine visits since it hit. Already, my colleagues are saying, 'This is great, let's do this after the pandemic ends.' We might have learned in a very scary way that this is a great way to deliver care to patients."[61]

[58] Carey B. The psychiatrist will see you online now. *The New York Times*. August 28, 2020.

[59] Shore JH, Schneck CD, Mishkind MC. Telepsychiatry and the coronavirus disease 2019 pandemic-current and future outcome of the rapid virtualization of psychiatric care. *JAMA Psychiatry*. May 11, 2020. 2020;77(12):1211–1212.

[60] Lees CW, Regueiro M, Mahadevan U, International Organization for the Study of Inflammatory Bowel Disease. Innovation in IBD care during the COVID-19 pandemic: Results of a global telemedicine survey by the International Organization for the Study of Inflammatory Bowel Disease. *Gastroenterology*. 2020. Sep;159(3):805.

[61] Seabrook J. The promise and the peril of virtual health care. *The New Yorker*. June 22, 2020.

In my own field of rheumatology, more than 80% of physicians in 64 countries had switched to telemedicine during the pandemic.[62] Almost 20% of their patients did not have access to video telehealth. Rheumatologists felt more comfortable using virtual visits with established patients compared to new patients. However, slightly less than 50% of rheumatologists agreed or strongly agreed that they were able to provide care efficiently with telemedicine and most thought that it was not time efficient.[63] In patients with established rheumatoid arthritis, those who opted for video telemedicine had a more favorable opinion about its general use, were seeing a rheumatologist who more often was using telemedicine, had higher disease activity scores, and had more visits with the rheumatologist in the preceding year.[64]

I can personally attest to the increasing use of telemedicine in cardiology. My cardiac pacemaker has been monitored remotely during the past year, and I have used my Apple Watch to back up my pulse readings, knowing that I haven't slipped back into atrial fibrillation. Neurologists have outlined a virtual cranial nerve examination and are able to measure visual acuity and balance virtually.[65] Oncology—with subspecialist expertise and teams that include genetic counselors, pathologists, palliative care specialists, social workers, and nutritionists—embraced the utility of telemedicine rounds.[66]

Inpatient and outpatient consultations during the pandemic were almost exclusively "E-consults," and this method of specialty consultation is likely to become increasingly adopted. E-consults increase patient and primary care access to specialists, decrease costs from travel, and have decreased three-quarters of in-person consultations when used appropriately.[67] In rheumatology even prior to the pandemic, E-consults for a positive antinuclear

[62] Mehta B, Jannat-Khah D, Fontana MA, Moezinia CJ, Mancuso CA, Bass AR, et al. Impact of COVID-19 on vulnerable patients with rheumatic disease: Results of a worldwide survey. *RMD Open*. October 6, 2020. doi: 10.1136/rmdopen-2020-001378.

[63] Singh JA, Richards JS, Chang E, Joseph A, Ng B. Management of rheumatic diseases during the COVID-19 pandemic: A National Veterans Affairs survey of rheumatologists. *Arthritis Care & Res*. October 15, 2020. https://doi.org/10.1002/acr.24487

[64] Ferucci ED, Holck P, Day GM, Choromanski TL, Freeman SL. Factors associated with use of telemedicine for follow-up of rheumatoid arthritis. *Arthritis Care & Res*. 2020;72:1404–1409.

[65] Grossman SN, Han SC, Balcer LJ, Kurzweil A, Weinberg H, Galetta SL, et al. Rapid implementation of virtual neurology in response to the COVID-19 pandemic. *Neurology*. June 16, 2020. 2020;94:24.

[66] West H. Telemedicine in oncology: Delivering on an overdue promise in the COVID-19 era. *Front Oncol*. September 25, 2020. doi: 10.3389/fonc.2020.578888.

[67] Ahmed S, Kelly YP, Behera TP, Kuye I, Blakey R, Goldstein SA, et al. Utility, appropriateness, and content of electronic consultations across medical subspecialties. *Ann Intern Med*. May 19, 2020;172:10. doi:10.7326/M19-3852.

antibody (ANA) tests were an effective way to address this common reason for a rheumatology consultation, thereby decreasing wait times for more appropriate in-person consultations.[68]

Now and in the Future

Telehealth use gradually leveled off during the later parts of 2020. From a peak of 70% virtual visits in July, virtual visits fell to 21% of all ambulatory visits in the United States in July 2020. Jessie DeVito, director of virtual care at Michigan Medicine, noted, "We're trying to right-size, but it's really hard because during the pandemic we switched to nearly 100% virtual in some clinical areas, and we know that's not realistic or sustainable."[69]

Before the COVID-19 pandemic, telemedicine had been a hard sell to US physicians. In 2016, 70% of large companies offered telehealth as part of their healthcare plans, but only 3% of workers used it.[70] A 2019 survey by the American Medical Association reported that only one-third of specialists and 40% of PCPs thought that virtual care would benefit their practices.[71] At a large Ohio primary care practice, those PCPs most resistant to virtual care tended to be in solo practice and had previously been resistant to implementation of electronic health records.[72]

Far and away, the most prominent concern with wide-scale adoption of telehealth is the inability to perform a detailed physical examination. Dr. Thomas Nash, an internist in New York City, complained, "Is it doable? Of course, it's doable. I'm doing it now. But I worry that it's going to delay a good exam and get in the way of deeper interactions between people and their doctors. Eyeball to eyeball is not a normal human interaction, right? A normal human interaction—you shift your body a little, you look to the left for a second, you gather your thoughts, you take a pause, which you

[68] Patel V, Stewart D, Horstman MJ. E-consults; an effective way to decrease wait times in rheumatology. *BMC Rheumatol*. October 15, 2020:4;54. doi: 10.1186/s41927-020-00152-5.

[69] Ross C. Telehealth grew wildly popular amid Covid-19. Now visits are plunging, forcing providers to recalibrate. *STAT*. September 1, 2020.

[70] Seabrook J. The promise and the peril of virtual health care. *The New Yorker*. June 22, 2020.

[71] Seabrook J. The promise and the peril of virtual health care. *The New Yorker*. June 22, 2020.

[72] Stone RL. How an Ohio-based physician organization overcame internal hurdles and launched a telehealth service as Covid-19 shutdowns loomed. *N Engl J Med*. October 8, 2020. https://catalyst.nejm.org/doi/full/10.1056/CAT.20.0515

really can't do in this compressed screen-to-screen interaction."[73] Dr. Marcin Chwistek, a palliative medicine specialist, worried, "Compared with the face-to-face interactions, the virtual interactions seem barren, devoid of the richness the personal contact brings. In a specialty like mine, where a lot depends on emotional connection with the patient and their caregivers, the virtual visits demanded more of me and yet felt a lot less fulfilling. And they all seemed to be plagued by annoying technical issues: a weak Wi-Fi signal, dropped connections, wrong phone numbers in the chart, malfunctioning headphones, or a broken phone camera. And what to do about the omnipresent background noise of a lawn mower? But there is no doubt that the virtual visit is a fundamental alteration to the patient–physician encounter."[74] Dr. Kevin Schulman, a hospitalist and economist at Stanford University, said, "I think there's going to be huge pressure to abandon all this."[75]

Not surprisingly, telemedicine has been much easier to implement and sustain in large healthcare organizations. Sharp Rees-Stealy (SRS), a 580-physician multispecialty group in San Diego, went from a few dozen telemedicine visits in February 2020 to 2,000 daily in March.[76] Initially with that switch the average telephone wait-time was 27 minutes, but they cut that back to 10 seconds within days by moving staff around to increase phone call capacity. High-resolution web cameras and other home equipment were provided, and staff were given "webside" manner training. As the pandemic stretched out to September 2020, SRS telemedicine accounted for 60% of all family and internal medicine visits with projections to continue to encompass about 30% of those visits in 2021 (Table 5.2).[77]

Small PCP practices in the United States and the United Kingdom never established extensive video care because of technological and financial barriers. The amount of time spent in virtual visits was generally longer than in-person, especially in smaller practices. There was a reluctance to invest in

---

[73] Seabrook J. The promise and the peril of virtual health care. *The New Yorker*. June 22, 2020.

[74] Chwistek M. "Are You Wearing Your White Coat?" Telemedicine in the time of pandemic. *JAMA* 2020;3242:149–150. doi:10.1001/jama.2020.10619.

[75] Span P. With red tape lifted, Dr. Zoom will see you now. *The New York Times*. May 8, 2020.

[76] Hrountas S, Bier AJ, Green S. A post Covid new normal: Developing fundamental changes for group medical practices. *N Engl J Med*. November 25, 2020. https://catalyst.nejm.org/doi/full/10.1056/CAT.20.0427

[77] Hrountas S, Bier AJ, Green S. A post Covid new normal: Developing fundamental changes for group medical practices. *N Engl J Med*. November 25, 2020. https://catalyst.nejm.org/doi/full/10.1056/CAT.20.0427

Table 5.2 Percent of Virtual Visits at Sharp Rees-Stealy

Medical Group	Week of 8/7/2020	Target for 2021
Family Medicine	60%	27%
Internal Medicine	60%	30%
Primary Care	52%	30%
Medical Specialties	36%	36%
Surgical Specialties	10%	9%
Pediatric Primary Care	16%	25%
All Patient Encounters	**38%**	**26%**

From: Hrountas S, Bier AJ, Green S. A post Covid new normal: Developing fundamental changes for group medical practices. *N Engl J Med.* November 25, 2020.

video conferencing without reassurances regarding the long-term financial viability of telemedicine.

Reimbursement for telemedicine during the latter part of 2020 varied from state to state and with insurance plans. Payers were concerned about fraud and abuse with telemedicine. However, there is no reason that telehealth auditing should be any more difficult than in-person audits. Sabrina Corlette, a research professor at Georgetown University, who did a report of how insurance companies responded to the pandemic, said, "Unless they are required to by the states or federal government, a lot of carriers will try to reimburse less for telehealth than an in-person visit."[78]

Benefits of widespread adoption of telemedicine for patients include the following:

- Greater access for patients, less disruptive
- After-hours telehealth reduces ER use
- Reduced cost for patients, less travel, less time away from work
- Good option for rural communities, patients with disabilities
- Easier access to specialists, medical information and education, clinical research

[78] Abelson R. Is telemedicine here to stay? *The New York Times.* August 3, 2020.

Benefits of widespread adoption of telemedicine for healthcare providers include the following:

- More flexibility, able to work at home
- Safer, such as during the pandemic
- Easier access to group management and education
- Fewer canceled appointments

Telemedicine could help alleviate critical care shortages since currently 50% of acute care hospitals have no ICU specialist on their staff.[79] This ability to care for patients across states via telehealth should continue. Telemedicine theoretically could lessen many of our healthcare inequities. It is ideally suited for serving rural communities, people with multiple chronic illnesses, and disabilities. It should make access to specialists easier and less costly. Patient portals and mobile health apps are "the primary touch points with the health care system . . . yet uptake has lagged among underserved populations, including patients of racial/ethnic minority groups, limited English proficiency, low socioeconomic status, older age, and low literacy."[80] For example, patients on Medicaid or with less than a high school diploma were twice as likely not to use patient portals.[81]

Equitable access to telemedicine has been difficult to implement during the pandemic. Primary care practices at the Univeristy of California, San Francisco, outlined a strategy to offset potential inequities of telemedicine in vulnerable populations such as those with limited digital literacy or access, rural residents, racial/ethnic minorities, older adults, and those with low income, limited health literacy, or limited English proficiency.[82] Recommendations to ensure equitable access to telemedicine included the following:

[79] Schoenberg R. Telehealth and the new choreography of "anywhere care." *STAT.* August 17, 2020.

[80] Rodriguez JA, Clark CR, Bates DW. Digital health equity as a necessity in the 21st century Cures Act era. *JAMA.* 2020 Jun 16;323(23):2381.

[81] Anthony DL, Campos-Castillo C, Lim PS. Who isn't using patient portals and why? Evidence and implications from a national sample of US adults. *Health Aff* (Millwood). 2018;37(12):1948–1954. doi: 10.1377/hlthaff.2018.05117.

[82] Nouri S, Khoong EC, Lyles CR, Karliner L. Addressing equity in telemedicine for chronic disease management during the Covid-19 pandemic. *N Engl J Med.* https://catalyst.nejm. May 4, 2020.

- Inform patients of free or reduced-cost broadband Internet
- Help patients obtain low-cost devices
- Ensure adequate language interpreters
- Help to enroll minority population in patient portals
- Offer telephone visit if video too difficult

Clinical suitability of telemedicine for an individual patient will vary based on the presenting symptoms and patient factors, such as poor cognition. A triage protocol for appropriate use of telemedicine in common patient scenarios was established at UCLA Health.[83] Chest pain would be extremely inappropriate for telemedicine, whereas depression or diabetes management would be considered very appropriate.

The most effective use of virtual healthcare in the future will require that providers are willing to adapt, as Dr. Amy Wheeler, a Massachusetts PCP, wrote in July 2020. "In the past, my encounters with patients during office visits usually included some portion of a physical exam, at least listening to their heart and lungs, so of course it's not the same thing to be staring at a video screen. A telemedicine visit feels like a shallow experience to some patients who want the 'real deal.' What I try to explain to my most stubborn patients is that up to 90% of my medical decisions are based on my asking questions, reviewing test results, and obtaining medical, family, and social histories—all things I can do virtually. There are even some surprising telemedicine benefits, such as having immediate access to a patient's pill bottles or glucose meter (no more 'I left it at home' excuses). I have actually been pleased by the quality of the care I can deliver through phone or video-based visits, even for chronic conditions like high blood pressure, high cholesterol, and diabetes."[84]

[83] Croymans D, Hurst I, Han M. Telehealth: The right care, at the right time, via the right medium. *N Engl J Med.* December 30, 2020. https://catalyst.nejm.org/doi/full/10.1056/CAT.20.0564

[84] Wheeler AE, My patients want the good old days of office visits. That's not happening any time soon. *STAT.* July 22, 2020.

6

COVID-19 Truths, Lies, and Consequences

Social Media Scourge

Healthcare professionals not only had to deal with the most lethal pandemic in a century, but they also had to counter unrelenting COVID misinformation and disinformation. Dr. Ryan Stanton, an emergency room physician in Kentucky, said a number of sick patients had waited until it was nearly too late to visit a hospital because they were convinced by what they had read online that COVID-19 was fake. "They thought it was just a ploy, a sham, a conspiracy. It just blew my mind that you can put these blinders on and ignore the facts."[1]

Drs. Seema Yasmin and Craig Spencer noted, "Purveyors of false news will always exist; for as long as there have been epidemics there have been snake-oil salespeople exploiting fear and peddling false hope. But Facebook enables these charlatans to thrive. Absent a concerted effort from Facebook to rework its algorithm in the best interests of public health—and not profit—we will continue to throw water on little fires of misinformation while an inferno blazes around us."[2] Even Yasmin and Spencer's medical coworkers weren't immune to all the misinformation. "Colleagues have confided in us that they believe the virus is manmade and diminishing in strength; others have asked us to invest money in Covid-19 'cures.' While we try, each day, to counter these dangerous falsehoods that circulate among our patients and our peers, our ability to counsel and provide care is diminished by a social

---

[1] Satariano A. Coronavirus doctors battle another scourge: Misinformation. *The New York Times*. August 17, 2020.
[2] Yasmin S, Spencer C. "But I saw it on Facebook": Hoaxes are making doctors' jobs harder. *The New York Times*. August 28, 2020.

network that bolsters distrust in science and medicine. Facebook is making it harder for us to do our jobs."[3]

During the first 6 months of the pandemic, 68,000 websites were registered with keywords related to COVID-19.[4] In April 2020, in the United States, the United Kingdom, France, Germany, and Italy, there were an estimated 460 million health falsehoods viewed on Facebook.[5] In Italy, from December 31, 2019, to April 30, 2020, 2 million fake news links related to COVID-19 were posted on the Internet, representing 23% of all COVID articles.[6]

The top 10 social media misinformation sites received four times as many Facebook views as the CDC, the WHO, and eight other leading health sites during April 2020.[7] A grouping of 42 Facebook pages were the main culprits of COVID misinformation and were being followed by 28 million people.[8] Websites such as GreenMedInfo and RealFarmacy were very successful at disseminating fake COVID news. One RealFarmacy article suggesting that COVID should be treated with colloidal silver was viewed 4.5 million times on Facebook.[9]

When personal protective equipment (PPE) was at a shortage, sham companies hoarded PPE supplies and sold them on their websites for outrageous prices. One auto body shop in New Jersey was "packed with enough medical equipment to outfit an entire hospital," and selling masks and gowns at a 700% markup.[10] A YouTube and Instagram video featuring a small-time actor claiming to have a pill that would ward off COVID was viewed more than 2 million times.[11] The Federal Trade Commission received more than

[3] Yasmin S, Spencer C. "But I saw it on Facebook": Hoaxes are making doctors' jobs harder. *The New York Times.* August 28, 2020.

[4] Ball P, Maxman A. The epic battle against coronavirus misinformation and conspiracy theories. *Nature.* May 27, 2020.

[5] Yasmin S, Spencer C. "But I saw it on Facebook": Hoaxes are making doctors' jobs harder. *The New York Times.* August 28, 2020.

[6] Moscadelli A, Albora G, Alberto Biamonte M, et al. Fake news and Covid-19 in Italy: Results of a quantitative observational study. *Int J Environ Res Public Health.* August 2020; 17(16):5850.

[7] Yasmin S, Spencer C. "But I saw it on Facebook": Hoaxes are making doctors' jobs harder. *The New York Times.* August 28, 2020.

[8] Yasmin S, Spencer C. "But I saw it on Facebook": Hoaxes are making doctors' jobs harder. *The New York Times.* August 28, 2020.

[9] Yasmin S, Spencer C. "But I saw it on Facebook": Hoaxes are making doctors' jobs harder. *The New York Times.* August 28, 2020.

[10] LaFraniere, S, Hamby C. Another thing to fear out there: Coronavirus scammers. *The New York Times.* April 5, 2020.

[11] Carrns A. Bogus vaccines. Fake testing sites. Virus frauds are flourishing. *The New York Times.* April 17, 2020.

18,000 COVID-related fraud complaints, with a reported loss of $9 million from January to April 15, 2020.[12] Phony drive-up websites accepted cash only to swab a person's cheek and run bogus tests while pseudo-medical clinics were giving intravenous vitamin C drips, claimed to bolster one's immunity. The single largest driver of misinformation about COVID-19 was President Trump. More than one-third of misinformation articles and posts on social media mentioned Trump.[13] At a press conference in April, Trump questioned whether "injections inside" the body of a disinfectant could kill the virus. Shortly thereafter, the CDC reported that 40% of US adults had misused cleaning products, including 19% putting bleach on foods, 18% applying household cleaners to their skin, and more than 5% drinking or inhaling disinfectant solutions.[14]

The Hydroxychloroquine Story

One of the most persistent COVID myths was that antimalarial drugs, in particular hydroxychloroquine, were effective treatments for COVID-19 infection. Here, too, President Trump played a pivotal role. The hydroxychloroqine-COVID-19 story provides a stark example of how half-truths, often touted by fringe scientists and championed by politicians and celebrities, became social media myths that mushroomed into COVID conspiracy theories.

In contrast to much of the COVID-related misinformation, there was some rationale to trying antimalarial medications for COVID-19. Like most rheumatologists, I had been using hydroxychloroquine for years in my patients with rheumatoid arthritis and systemic lupus erythematosus and was aware of its modest immune and anti-inflammatory effect and relative safety. I was not surprised that it was being investigated in early clinical trials in patients with COVID-19 infection, spurred by two small studies from China suggesting that it may have some efficacy. By early March, the antimalarials were the subject of more than 100 worldwide COVID-19 clinical trials,

[12] Carrns A. Bogus vaccines. Fake testing sites. Virus frauds are flourishing. *The New York Times.* April 17, 2020.
[13] Stolberg SG, Weiland N. Study finds single largest driver of coronavirus misinformation: Trump. *The New York Times.* September 30, 2020.
[14] Joseph A. Some Americans are misusing cleaning products—including drinking them—in effort to kill coronavirus. *STAT.* June 5, 2020.

by far more than any other medication. This interest in using antimalarials to treat COVID-19 was sparked by a controversial French microbiologist, Didier Raoult, who posted a short, triumphant video on YouTube titled "Coronavirus: Game Over!"[15] This was based on the two small studies from China and Raoult's own study, from which he claimed, "a 100 percent cure rate."[16]

Raoult's study consisted of just 36 patients, at various stages of COVID-19 infection, 14 treated with hydroxychloroquine, 6 with hydroxychloroquine and azithromycin, and 16 controls. He claimed that most of the patients on the medications cleared the virus after just 6 days, including all six given the two drugs, compared to just a few of the controls. There were no data provided on patient symptoms or on their eventual clinical outcome. Six of the patients that had been started on hydroxychloroquine were "lost to follow-up" with no results provided. Some of the subjects said to be cleared of the virus were later found to be carrying the virus 2 days after the study.

Raoult admitted that this small study was not done in a controlled, blinded fashion but asserted that randomized, controlled trials were "not only unnecessary but unethical."[17] Subsequent uncontrolled, larger studies by Raoult and coworkers were touted as confirming his conclusion that the two drugs effectively lowered COVID-19 viral load.[18] These studies had identical methodological errors and subsequently were discounted by the journal that published them.[19]

On March 16, Laura Ingraham, at Fox News, introduced a Long Island attorney, Gregory Rigano, with the leading question, "What if there's already a cheap and widely available medication, that's on the market, to treat the virus? Well, according to a new study, there is such a drug. It's called chloroquine."[20] Rigano, falsely saying that he was an adviser to Stanford

---

[15] Sayare S. He was a science star. Then he promoted a questionable cure for Covid-19. *The New York Times.* May 12, 2020.

[16] Sayare S. He was a science star. Then he promoted a questionable cure for Covid-19. *The New York Times.* May 12, 2020.

[17] Sayare S. He was a science star. Then he promoted a questionable cure for Covid-19. *The New York Times.* May 12, 2020.

[18] Million M, Lagier J-C, Gautret P, et al. Early treatment of COVID-19 patients with hydroxychloroquine and azithromycin: A retrospective analysis of 1061 cases in Marseille, France. *Travel Med Infect Dis.* May–June 2020. 2020;35:101738.

[19] Machiels JD, Bleeker-Rovers CP, Heine RT, et al. Reply to Gautret et al: Hydroxychloroquine sulfate and azithromycin for COVID-19: What is the evidence and what are the risks? *Int J Antimicrob Agents.* July 2020. 2020;56:106056.

[20] Sayare S. He was a science star. Then he promoted a questionable cure for Covid-19. *The New York Times.* May 12, 2020.

Medical School, had self-published a review of Raoult's early results, noting that "one of the most eminent infectious-disease specialists in the whole world . . . demonstrated that within a matter of six days, the patients taking hydroxychloroquine tested negative for coronavirus, for Covid-19. We have a strong reason to believe that a preventative dose of hydroxychloroquine is going to prevent the virus from attaching to the body, and just get rid of it completely."[21] Raoult had agreed to share his results with Rigano and allowed these unsubstantiated results to be posted on Twitter before they were published. That week Rigano appeared on Tucker Carlson's Fox show, Raoult was a guest on "Dr. Oz," and Trump tweeted that the results were "very, very encouraging and I think it could be something really incredible."[22]

By the evening of March 19, there were 32,000 first-time prescriptions written for the antimalarials, 46 times greater than the usual daily average.[23] More than 40,000 healthcare professionals became first-time prescribers of antimalarial medications, mainly primary care physicians who had never prescribed an antimalarial medication in the past. Carmen Catizone, executive director of the National Association of Boards of Pharmacy, said that the resultant hydroxychloroquine drug shortages "put patients at risk who depend on these medications. The fact that people reacted to what the White House said in such a way—in the 35 years I've been in pharmacy and pharmacy regulation, I've never seen that before."[24] The following day, Trump tweeted that he was taking hydroxychloroquine as preventative medicine and advising the public to do the same: "What do you have to lose? I really think they should take it. But it's their choice. And it's their doctor's choice or the doctors in the hospital. But hydroxychloroquine. Try it, if you'd like."[25] The next day Google searches in the United States related to the purchase of hydroxychloroquine increased exponentially.[26]

[21] Sayare S. He was a science star. Then he promoted a questionable cure for Covid-19. *The New York Times.* May 12, 2020.

[22] Sayare S. He was a science star. Then he promoted a questionable cure for Covid-19. *The New York Times.* May 12, 2020.

[23] Gabler E, Keller MH. Prescriptions surged as Trump praised drugs in coronavirus fight. *The New York Times.* April 25, 2020.

[24] Gabler E, Keller MH. Prescriptions surged as Trump praised drugs in coronavirus fight. *The New York Times.* April 25, 2020.

[25] Torres. OL Trump keeps putting the lives of Lupus patients at risk. *The New York Times.* April 6, 2020.

[26] Liu M, Caputi TL, Dredze M, et al. Internet searches for unproven COVID-19 therapies in the United States. *JAMA.* April 29, 2020. 2020;180(8):1116–1118.

On March 28, 2020, the FDA granted a waiver, referred to as an Emergency Use Authorization (EUA), "for emergency use of oral formulations of chloroquine phosphate and hydroxychloroquine sulfate for the treatment of COVID-19."[27] Within days, most US hospitals and many clinical practices were prescribing antimalarials to patients with suspected or confirmed COVID-19 infection. In the single month of March 2020, 300,000 new patients in the United States received hydroxychloroquine, including 93,000 who also received a new prescription for azithromycin, which some thought augmented its therapeutic benefit.[28]

Clinicians throughout the country immediately expressed concern about this widespread use of antimalarial medications with little evidence for its efficacy. Yet many physicians were writing prescriptions for themselves or family members. Dr. Tamar Barlam, chief of infectious disease at Boston Medical Center, said, "The issue for me that's disturbing is that people are getting their own prescriptions . . . doctors or dentists are writing themselves large prescriptions of the drugs, and doing it for themselves and family. If there's hoarding, that is just going to be a big problem, and that is something that pharmacies and the healthcare system need to put a stop to pretty quickly."[29]

Peter Navarro, Trump's trade adviser, worked with the Federal Emergency Management Agency to push 19 million pills of hydroxychloroquine from the nation's stockpiles to 14 coronavirus hot zones, stoking the hydroxychloroquine fervor by asking, "Has the media's war of hysteria on hydroxychloroquine killed people?"[30] Dr. Steven Nissen, a cardiologist at the Cleveland Clinic, responded, "Peter Navarro is not a scientist, he is the president's trade representative. He should not be advising the public on matters of health."[31]

[27] Letter to Dr. Rick Bright re: Request for Emergency Use Authorization for use of chloroquine phosphate or hydroxychloroquine sulfate supplied from the strategic national stockpile for treatment of 2019 coronavirus disease. March 28, 2020. Accessed August 3, 2020. https://www.fda.gov/media/136534/download

[28] Shehab N, Lovegrove M, Budnitz DS. US hydroxychloroquine, chloroquine, and azithromycin outpatient prescription trends, October 2019 through March 2020. *JAMA Intern Med.* July 6, 2020;180(10):1384–1386.

[29] Rowland C. As Trump touts an unproven coronavirus treatment, supplies evaporate for patients who need these drugs. *The Washington Post.* March 23, 2020.

[30] Herper M. A flawed Covid-19 study gets the White House's attention—and the FDA may pay the price. *STAT.* July 8, 2020.

[31] Herper M. A flawed Covid-19 study gets the White House's attention—and the FDA may pay the price. *STAT.* July 8, 2020.

In early April, a Southern California doctor, Jennings Ryan Staley, was arrested and charged with mail fraud, for selling "Covid-19 treatment packs that were a 100% cure."[32] Staley, the owner of the Skinny Beach Med Spa in San Diego, provided medication packs containing hydroxychloroquine and azithromycin, as well as anti-anxiety and sleeping medications, billed as "a concierge medicine experience" at $3,995 for a family of four. Staley claimed, "It's preventative and curative. It's hard to believe, it's almost too good to be true. But it's a remarkable clinical phenomenon."[33] Staley's lawyer defended his client: "The same executive branch that has been touting these two medications for weeks has now turned around and criminally charged an Iraq veteran, Dr. Staley, no criminal record, for doing exactly the same thing that the administration's been doing this whole time."[34]

During the next 2 months, a number of studies confirmed that hydroxychloroquine alone or in combination with azithromycin was not effective in patients with COVID-19 infection.[35] The largest study, part of the UK RECOVERY trial, compared 1,542 patients treated with high doses of hydroxychloroquine to 3,132 control patients and found no morbidity or mortality efficacy.[36] On June 15, the FDA revoked the emergency approval of antimalarial drugs. Senator Ron Wyden of Oregon noted, "The F.D.A. withdrew an emergency use authorization that never should have been issued in the first place. By ignoring science and caving to political pressure from the White House, the F.D.A. stoked false hope and put American lives in danger, while damaging the agency's reputation in the process."[37] Peter Navarro pushed back: "This is a Deep State blindside by bureaucrats who hate the administration they work for more than they're concerned about

---

[32] Ortiz A. Doctor charged with fraud after U.S. says he sold treatment as "100 percent" cure for Covid-19. *The New York Times.* April 17, 2020.

[33] Ortiz A. Doctor charged with fraud after U.S. says he sold treatment as "100 percent" cure for Covid-19. *The New York Times.* April 17, 2020.

[34] Ortiz A. Doctor charged with fraud after U.S. says he sold treatment as "100 percent" cure for Covid-19. *The New York Times.* April 17, 2020.

[35] Rosenberg ES, Dufort EM, Udo T, et al. Association of treatment with Hydroxychloroquine or Azithromycin with in-hospital mortality in patients with COVID-19 in New York State. *JAMA.* June 23 2020;323:2493–2502.

[36] Torjesen I. Covid-19: Hydroxychloroquine does not benefit hospitalized patients, UK trial finds. *BMJ.* 22020;369.

[37] Thomas K. F.D.A. revokes emergency approval of malaria drugs promoted by Trump. *The New York Times.* June 15, 2020.

saving American lives."[38] Sixty-three million tablets of hydroxychloroquine remained sitting unused.

Despite medical experts' consensus that hydroxychloroquine is ineffective, Trump and other politicians persisted in posting pseudoscientific blogs about the drug. On July 28, a group calling themselves America's Frontline Doctors posted a video of themselves in front of the Supreme Court claiming that hydroxychloroquine is a "cure for Covid" and adding that wearing masks was a hoax.[39] Within 6 hours, President Trump and Donald Trump Jr. retweeted the video, and then it was live-streamed by Brietbart and subsequently viewed more than 14 million times until finally removed by Facebook, YouTube, and Twitter.[40] This video featured Dr. Stella Immanuel, a physician in Texas, who runs a church called Fire Power Ministries. Dr. Immanuel also suggested that many gynecological problems, including endometriosis, are caused by people having sex with witches and demons during their dreams. When asked about Immanuel and her group, Trump commented: "I think they're very respected doctors. There was a woman who was spectacular. I thought she was very impressive, in the sense that, from where she came—I don't know what country she comes from—but she said that she's had tremendous success with hundreds of different patients . . . and they took her voice off. I don't know why they took her off. Maybe they had a good reason, maybe they didn't. I thought her voice was an important voice, but I know nothing about her."[41]

As of September 10, 2020, 24% of Americans still thought that hydroxychloroquine was an effective treatment for COVID, including 51% of Republicans compared to 8% of Democrats.[42] Dr. Michael Saag wrote in *JAMA* on November 9, 2020, "The number of articles in the peer reviewed literature over the last several months that have consistently and convincingly demonstrated the lack of efficacy of a highly hyped 'cure' for COVID-19

---

[38] Stolberg SG. A mad scramble to stock millions of malaria drugs, likely for nothing. *The New York Times.* June 16, 2020.

[39] Frenkel S, Alba D. Misleading virus video, pushed by the Trumps, spreads online. *The New York Times.* July 28, 2020.

[40] Andrews TM, Paquette D. Trump retweeted a video with false Covid-19 claims. *The Washington Post.* July 29, 2020.

[41] Andrews TM, Paquette D. Trump retweeted a video with false Covid-19 claims. *The Washington Post.* July 29, 2020.

[42] Hamel l, Kearney A, Kirzinger A, Lopes L, Munana C, Brodie M. KFF Health Tracking Poll—September 2020: Top Issues in 2020 Election, the role of misinformation, and views on a potential coronavirus vaccine. Kaiser Foundation Health Tracker. September 10, 2020.

represent the consequence of the irresponsible infusion of politics into the world of scientific evidence and discourse. For other potential therapies or interventions for COVID-19 (or any other diseases), this should not happen again."[43]

Conspiracy Theories and Anti-Vaccination Movements

At least the hydroxychloroquine rumors and myths began in the context of potential medical rationale. In contrast, the most prominent COVID conspiracy theories have no semblance of science. Conspiracy theories are a source of disinformation, defined as organized falsehoods intended to deceive. Many of the COVID-related conspiracy theories have been generated by the anti-vaccination movement whose messages reached 60–100 million online viewers.[44]

The video "Plandemic," posted on social media on May 4, 2020, featured a discredited research scientist, Dr. Judy Mikovits, who claimed that public health experts misled the public about the virus. She asserted that COVID-19 was the result of contaminated animal vaccine experiments, and that Big Pharma, wealthy people, and "corrupt mainstream scientists" intentionally spread the virus so the general population would be forced to vaccinate.[45] Within 24 hours, a Facebook group dedicated to QAnon posted the video to its 25,000 members with the caption, "Exclusive Content, Must Watch," and before it was taken down by YouTube, Facebook, Twitter, and Instagram, "Plandemic" was viewed more than 8 million times.[46] Once again President Trump and Donald Trump Jr., as well as Kelli Ward, the Arizona Republican Party chairwoman, shared links to the video.[47]

---

[43] Saag MS. Misguided use of hydroxychloroquine for COVID-19. *JAMA*. November 9, 2020. 2020;324(21):2161–2162.

[44] Editors. The COVID-19 infodemic. *The Lancet Infectious Disease*. August 2020;20(8):875.

[45] Frankel S, Decker B, Alba D. How the "Plandemic" movie and its falsehood spread widely online. *The New York Times*. May 20, 2020.

[46] Frankel S, Decker B, Alba D. How the "Plandemic" movie and its falsehood spread widely online. *The New York Times*. May 20, 2020.

[47] Fisher M, Weiner R. With little clarity on coronavirus, Americans crowdsource how to live in a pandemic. *The Washington Post*. July 20, 2020.

I was familiar with Mikovitz since I had reviewed her 2009 research paper asserting that chronic fatigue syndrome was caused by a retrovirus.[48] That paper was subsequently retracted from *Science* after it was shown to be fraudulent and scientifically invalid.[49] Mikovitz was fired from her job at the privately funded Whittemore Peterson Institute and arrested for theft of research data and materials. In the film, Mikovitz ranted about government conspiracies and attacked Dr. Anthony Fauci, whom she falsely claimed barred her from NIH property.[50] Dr. Peter J. Hotez, Dean of the National School of Tropical Medicine at Baylor College of Medicine, said that Mikovitz's rise as the darling of anti-vaccine groups had "taken a new ominous twist with the coronavirus. They've now aligned themselves with far-right groups and their weapons of choice are YouTube, Facebook, and Amazon."[51]

In June 2020, 10% of Facebook pages regarding vaccines were dedicated to anti-vaccine theories.[52] One of the leaders of the anti-vax movement is Andrew Wakefield, who had published the fraudulent study that the MMR vaccine was linked to autism and subsequently had his medical license revoked. Wakefield claimed, "One of the main tenets of the marketing of mandatory vaccination has been fear. And never have we seen fear exploited in the way that we do now with the coronavirus infection. I think what we have reached is a situation where— I hope we've reached a situation where—the public are now sufficiently skeptical."[53] Bill Gates, despite spending much of his time and money on COVID-19 technology, treatment, and vaccines, was continuously targeted by anti-vax groups. Robert F. Kennedy Jr., a strong anti-vaccination activist, claimed that Gates was using the vaccine as a means to monitor people via an injected microchip designed to track and control people's actions.[54] Roger Stone, Trump's former advisor, said on radio that he

[48] Shepherd K. Who is Judy Mikovits in "Plandemic," the coronavirus conspiracy video just banned from social media? *The Washington Post*. May 8, 2020.

[49] Neil SJD, Campbell EM. Fake science: XMRV, COVID-19, and the toxic legacy of Dr. Judy Mikovitz. *AIDS Res Hum Retroviruses*. July 2020;36:545–549.

[50] Lytvynenko J. The "Plandemic" video has exploded online—and it is filled with falsehoods. *BuzzFeed*. May 7, 2020.

[51] Alba D. Virus conspiracists elevate a new champion. *The New York Times*. May 9, 2020.

[52] Cornwell W. Just 50% of Americans plan to get a COVID-19 vaccine. *Science*. June 30, 2020.

[53] Jamison P. Anti-vaccination leaders seize on coronavirus to push resistance to inoculation. *The Washington Post*. May 5, 2020.

[54] Jamison P. Anti-vaccination leaders seize on coronavirus to push resistance to inoculation. *The Washington Post*. May 5, 2020.

would never trust a vaccine funded by Gates and that interview was covered without any disclaimer by the *New York Post*, then shared or commented on by 1 million Facebook posts.[55] A popular theory suggested that Dr. Fauci, like Gates, was exaggerating COVID deaths, and Facebook attacks on Fauci spiked after Trump retweeted a Twitter post "Time to Fire Fauci."[56]

During the early stages of the pandemic, worry about infection slowed rates of routine immunizations. In the United States there was a decline of 2.5 million routine vaccinations from January through April 2020 compared to the previous year, and it was estimated that 117 million children in 37 countries had not yet received their scheduled measles vaccinations.[57] Erica DeWald, director of advocacy at the nonprofit group Vaccinate Your Family, countered, "I've watched the leaders of the anti-vaccine movement scare parents for years. And in this moment, when parents are more scared than ever, they're profiting off of it. Basically, the anti-vaccine leaders are telling their followers, 'This is not real, this is not a concern for you, if you're healthy, if you eat well, if you sleep enough, you will be fine. And this is once again a gateway for the government to force vaccines on to you and your children.'"

Vaccine mistrust has been on the rise in the United States for years and crosses party and demographic lines. The "warp speed" campaign aggravated concerns over haste to get the COVID vaccine out. Black Americans have been notably wary, partly stemming from the notorious Tuskegee experiments, in which Black men were purposely not treated for syphilis without their consent. In July, only 32% of Black Americans said that they would definitely get a COVID vaccine. Dr. Fauci commented, "It is of great concern to me. If there's anyone you want to get vaccinated, and anyone for whom vaccination would be most beneficial, it would be for the people [anti-vaccination activists] are trying to influence not to get vaccinated."[58]

More than 30% of Americans expressed belief in at least one of the conspiracy theories about the origin of the COVID pandemic.[59] Conspiracy

[55] Ball P, Maxmen A. The epic battle against coronavirus misinformation and conspiracy theories. *Nature.* May 27, 2020.

[56] White House denies Trump is considering firing Fauci despite his retweet of a hashtag calling for his ouster. https://www.washingtonpost.com/nation/2020/04/13/trump-fire-fauci-coronavirus/. Accessed June 11, 2020.

[57] Stephenson J. Sharp drop in routine vaccinations for US children amid COVID-19 pandemic. *JAMA Network.* May 12, 2020.

[58] Jamison P. Anti-vaccination leaders seize on coronavirus to push resistance to inoculation. *The Washington Post.* May 5, 2020.

[59] Enders AM, Uscinski JE. Conspiracy theories run rampant when people feel helpless. Like now. *The Washington Post.* May 5, 2020.

theories explode during times of crisis and uncertainty, generated by organized groups for political and financial gain. Mike Wood, a psychologist and expert on belief in conspiracy theories who studied the spread of misinformation during the Zika outbreak in 2016, said, "There are people who believe one conspiracy theory or another because it fits their political beliefs, and there are some people for whom conspiracy theories are their beliefs. For those people, the specifics of the conspiracy theory don't matter all that much. A lot of times, these are recycled from earlier conspiracy theories. In a pandemic, there's immediately going to be conspiracy theories that the virus is either harmless, a bioweapon that's going to kill everybody, or an excuse for the government to give a vaccine that is going to kill everybody."[60] In mid-December 2020, 30% of Americans said they would definitely or probably not get the vaccine even if it was deemed safe and free.[61] This included 35% of Black adults, 42% of Republicans, and 33% of essential workers.

Ross McKinney Jr., a virologist and chief scientific officer for the Association of American Medical Colleges, noted that disregarding expert opinion has become more prominent during the COVID pandemic than ever before. "When SARS hit in 2003 and the H1N1 flu virus erupted in 2009, we turned to the professionals and listened to the CDC, to people who have established reputations for being credible and straightforward. Now, between the lack of certainty about how this virus will behave over time, the country's sharp political polarization, and the widespread denigration of expertise in many fields, people feel lost. This time, it's possible that people may not come around to believing the experts. We as a culture are in the midst of an evolution in how we gather and consider information, and this epidemic came at exactly the wrong time in that evolution. You want to rely on authoritative figures who do this kind of work. But with this flood of information, we all have to realize what our own biases are. Do you want to believe something because it confirms your hopes?"[62]

[60] Andrews TM. Why dangerous conspiracy theories about the virus spread so fast—and how they can be stopped. *The Washington Post.* May 1, 2020.

[61] Hamel L, Kirzinger A, Munana C, Brodie M. KFF COVID-19 vaccine monitor: December 2020. KFF. Accessed December 15, 2020.

[62] Fisher M, Weiner R. With little clarity on coronavirus, Americans crowdsource how to live in a pandemic. *The Washington Post.* July 20, 2020.

Denigrating Public Health and Science

Both the CDC and the FDA made a number of strategic errors and basically botched the initial rollout of US COVID-19 testing. On February 4, just a few days after Germany reported the first test for COVID-19, the CDC obtained emergency approval of its own test from the FDA and then began shipping out kits to 100 public health labs across the country. The CDC test consisted of three genetic probes, two for COVID-19 and a third to detect other coronaviruses. That third probe was quickly found faulty, triggering false-positive results. Scott Becker the executive director of the Association of Public Health Laboratories, said, "On the morning of February 8th, my cellphone began blowing up with messages from member labs. I started to see this string of problems, and I thought, 'Oh, my God, this can't be happening.' If this test had a problem, we were weeks behind and we were not going to be able to contain this."[63]

At the time, the World Health Organization (WHO) had developed a reliable test so the CDC could have pivoted to that test or used university and private labs to develop their own tests. Alex Azar at the Department of Health and Human Services (HHS) made the FDA the gatekeeper for any final COVID-19 test approval, so private and university labs testing development was difficult. Kathleen Sebelius, Obama's HHS secretary, said "It's a real problem that we didn't immediately pivot to the WHO test, which we knew was working very well. We could have purchased a lot of those and pushed them out. We could have opened up the private-lab capacity. And we didn't do any of that."[64] The CDC could have simply eliminated the third probe from their COVID test which is exactly what they did 1 month later. A testing bottleneck led to extreme rationing of tests for months in the United States. *The New York Times* commented, "The result was a lost month, when the world's richest country—armed with some of the most highly trained scientists and infectious disease specialists—squandered its best chance of containing the virus's spread. Instead, Americans were left largely blind to the scale of a looming public health catastrophe."[65]

---

[63] Dickinson T. The four men responsible for America's COVID-19 test disaster. *Rolling Stone*. May 10, 2020.
[64] Dickinson T. The four men responsible for America's COVID-19 test disaster. *Rolling Stone*. May 10, 2020.
[65] Shear MD, Goodnough A, Kaplan S, Fink S, Thomas K, Weiland N. The lost month: How a failure to test blinded the U.S. to Covid-19. *The New York Times*. March 28, 2020.

On February 25, 2020, Nancy Messonnier, the CDC's director of the National Center of Immunization and Respiratory Diseases, warned of a wide COVID-19 outbreak in the United States: "It's not so much a question of if this will happen anymore, but rather a question of exactly when and disruption to everyday life may be severe."[66] That same week, Trump insisted that infections had peaked, "We have a total of 15 people diagnosed with it and within a couple of days is going to be down close to zero,"[67] and added that Democrats were "politicizing the coronavirus, it's a hoax and we have lost nobody."[68] Following Messonnier's predictions, Trump exploded, took Azar out of the COVID task force lead, installed Mike Pence, and permanently silenced Messonnier. Months later, Kyle McGowan, CDC chief of staff at the time, defended Messonnier, "There's not a single thing that she said that didn't come true. Is it more important to have her telling the world and the American public what to be prepared for, or is it just to say, 'All is well?' It's demoralizing to spend your entire career preparing for this moment, preparing for a pandemic like this. And then not be able to fully do your job. They need to be allowed to lead."[69]

On February 14, Alex Greninger, assistant director of the University of Washington's clinical virology lab, described the bureaucratic hurdles at the FDA. "The most pernicious effect of the current regulatory environment is that it kneecaps our ability for preparedness should a true emergency emerge."[70] Rick Bright, at the time the director of HHS's Biomedical Advanced Research and Development Authority (BARDA), warned Azar about the global threat but said that Azar was "downplaying this catastrophic threat."[71]

Even before COVID, public health experts voiced concern when Dr. Robert Redfield was appointed CDC commissioner by Trump in 2018.

---

[66] Dickinson T. The four men responsible for America's COVID-19 test disaster. *Rolling Stone*. May 10, 2020.

[67] Dickinson T. The four men responsible for America's COVID-19 test disaster. *Rolling Stone*. May 10, 2020.

[68] *Totally under control*. Alex Gibney, director. NEON. Accessed October 13, 2020.

[69] Weiland N. "Like a hand grasping": Trump appointees describe the crushing of the C.D.C. *The New York Times*. December 16, 2020.

[70] Boburg S, O'Harrow R Jr, Satija N, Goldstein A. Inside the coronavirus testing failure: Alarm and dismay among the scientists who sought to help. *The Washington Post*. April 3, 2020.

[71] Dickinson T. The four men responsible for America's COVID-19 disaster. *Rolling Stone*. May 10, 2020.

On February 29, at a White House briefing, Redfield told Americans, "the risk at this time is low. The American public need to go on with their normal lives."[72] That was the same day that the FDA finally loosened its restriction on labs outside the CDC testing for COVID-19. Dr. Ashish Jha, director of the Harvard Global Health Institute, said in April, "As we struggle our way through this, an essential element is missing: strong, effective leadership from the Centers for Disease Control and Prevention, the premier public health agency in the world. During this pandemic, when accurate, timely, nationwide information is the lifeblood of our response, the CDC has largely disappeared."[73] With lack of funding, the CDC's information tracking systems had become antiquated and "The CDC could not produce accurate counts of how many people were being tested, compile complete demographic information on confirmed cases or even keep timely tallies of deaths. Backups on at least some of these systems are made on recordable DVDs, a technology that was state-of-the-art in the late 1990s."[74]

In early March, the Department of Health and Human Services stopped giving the CDC clearance to hold press briefings. Subsequently the CDC went 95 days without holding a COVID-19 related press conference. In April and May, the administration consistently interfered with the CDC recommendations urging schools, houses of worship, day camps, restaurants, and child-care centers to move slowly and only with specific precautions. The CDC recommended in May that church choirs be suspended or greatly limited, but Pence removed that guideline.[75] In July, a document targeting the importance of school reopening was dropped into the CDC website by the Department of Health and Human Services. Education Secretary Betsy DeVos said that the CDC guidelines were an impediment to rational reopening of schools. Mike Pence told reporters, "The president said today we just don't want the guidance to be too tough. And that's the reason next week the CDC is going to be issuing a new set of tools."[76]

---

[72] Dickinson T. The four men responsible for America's COVID-19 disaster. *Rolling Stone.* May 10, 2020.

[73] Jha AK. We need the real CDC back, and we need it now. *STAT.* April 29, 2020.

[74] Lipton E, Goodnough A, Shear MD, Twohey M, Mandavilli A, Fink S, Walker M. The C.D.C. waited 'its entire existence for this moment.' What went wrong? *The New York Times.* June 3, 2020.

[75] Branswell H. As controversies swirl, CDC director is seen as allowing agency to buckle to political influence. *STAT.* September 16, 2020.

[76] Sun LH, Dawsey J. CDC feels pressure from Trump as rift grows over coronavirus response. *The Washington Post.* July 9, 2020.

Mark Rosenberg, the first director of the CDC's National Center for Injury Prevention and Control, worried, "They worked on the school guidelines for months. Around the clock, 24/7, they were working to get the best scientific guidance for the country. And then . . . the White House stuck an introduction on the front of it on the CDC website that said: 'The most important thing is for kids to go back to school.' That wasn't written by CDC. That wasn't anything CDC people wanted to say. A reputation that takes 75 years to build can be destroyed in four months. That's horrifying."[77] Trump and colleagues referred to CDC scientists as disloyal liberals and members of the "deep state." Lawrence Gostin, a former CDC official, said, "Public health is politics. But this is different. It's criticizing its public health agencies in public. It's rejecting guidelines it puts out. It tells them you can't even put guidelines out. I would expect the CDC to coordinate with the White House. But this is not teamwork. This is not coordination. This is confrontation."[78]

Four former CDC directors commented, "Through last week, and into Monday, the administration continued to cast public doubt on the agency's recommendations and role in informing and guiding the nation's pandemic response. We're seeing the terrible effect of undermining the CDC play out in our population. Willful disregard for public health guidelines is, unsurprisingly, leading to a sharp rise in infections and deaths. Trying to fight this pandemic while subverting scientific expertise is like fighting blindfolded. How well and how quickly we adhere to the advice of public health experts at the CDC will determine whether, how soon and how safely our schools can reopen."[79] Kyle McGowan, CDC chief of staff and a Trump appointee, said, "Everyone wants to describe the day that the light switch flipped and the CDC was sidelined. It didn't happen that way. It was more like a hand grasping something, and it slowly closes, closes, closes, closes until you realize that, middle of the summer, it has a complete grasp on everything at the CDC."[80]

[77] Branswell H. As controversies swirl, CDC director is seen as allowing agency to buckle to political influence. *STAT*. September 16, 2020.

[78] Lipton E, Goodnough A, Shear MD, Twohey M, Mandavilli A, Fink S, Walker M. The CDC waited 'its entire existence for this moment.' What went wrong? *The New York Times*. June 3, 2020.

[79] Frieden T, Koplan J, Satcher D, Besser R. We ran the CDC. No president ever politicized its science the way Trump has. *The Washington Post*. July 14, 2020.

[80] Weiland N. "Like a hand grasping": Trump appointees describe the crushing of the C.D.C. *The New York Times*. December 16, 2020.

In late August the FDA gave emergency authorization for the use of convalescent plasma to treat COVID-19, Trump calling the treatment, a "very historic breakthrough."[81] That same day, Hahn badly misconstrued a Mayo Clinic study by saying that these researchers had found a 35% survival benefit with the use of convalescent plasma. Trump called it "a tremendous number" and Azar said, "I don't want you to gloss over this number."[82] Hahn told reporters, "Many of you know I was a cancer doctor before I became FDA commissioner. And a 35% improvement in survival is a pretty substantial clinical benefit."[83] The problem was Hahn's faulty statistics since the study showed a 3%–5% improvement. Bill Gates was harsh in his criticism of Hahn: "This is third grade math. I mean, are you kidding? The head of the FDA got up and said it was a 35% death reduction where it's not even a 3% reduction based on just a tiny little subset that was nonstatistical. This is unheard of."[84] A few days later Hahn admitted that his statement was misleading.

In late August, the CDC declared that people who had been in close contact with an infected person, "do not necessarily need a test" if they don't have symptoms. After a huge outcry from scientists and physicians, a few days later this was revised to "testing may be considered for all close contacts of confirmed or probable Covid-19 patients."[85] The CDC kept changing its position on airborne viral transmission, most notably on small particle aerosol spread, which was added to its guidelines, then quickly removed and then reinserted in late September.[86]

In September, administration officials attempted to revise or delay publication of scientific reports in the CDC's publication, *Morbidity and Mortality Reports (MMWR)*.[87] *MMWR* is the United States's most trusted source to track infections and infection control and has never before been interfered

[81] McGinley L, Abutaleb Y, Dawsey J, Johnson CY. Inside Trumps's pressure campaign on federal scientists over a covid-19 treatment. *The Washington Post*. August 30, 2020.

[82] Thomas K, Fink S. F.D.A. "grossly misrepresented" blood plasma data, scientists say. *The New York Times*. August 24, 2020.

[83] Branswell H. Bill Gates slams "shocking" U.S. response to Covid-19 pandemic. *STAT*. September 4, 2020.

[84] Branswell H. Bill Gates slams 'shocking' U.S. response to Covid-19 pandemic. *STAT*. September 4, 2020.

[85] Stolberg SG. C.D.C.'s "clarification" on coronavirus testing offers more confusion. *The New York Times*. August 27, 2020.

[86] Elfrink T, Guarino B, Mooney C. CDC reverses itself and says guidelines it posted on coronavirus airborne transmission were wrong. *The Washington Post*. September 21, 2020.

[87] Weiland W, Stolberg SG, Goodnough A. Political appointees meddled in C.D.C.'s "holiest of the holy." *The New York Times*. September 12, 2020.

with by political appointees. Dr. William Schaffner, an infectious disease specialist at Vanderbilt University and a member of the external editorial board of the *MMWR*, commented that "The *MMWR* had an unblemished reputation as being accurate, objective and science-based, free from political influence and such political interference undermines the credibility of not only the *MMWR*, but of the C.D.C. And the C.D.C.'s credibility has been tarnished throughout Covid already."[88]

That month Trump contradicted Redfield's message to Congress that a vaccine would not be widely distributed until the middle of 2021, Trump saying that Redfield was "confused."[89] Then on September 26, after Redfield said that about 90% of Americans remain vulnerable to COVID-19, Dr. Scott Atlas, Trump's new pandemic adviser, who had no public health background, told reporters that Redfield was wrong and replied, "You're supposed to believe the science and I'm telling you the science."[90] Atlas also helped Trump reissue a disguised call for "herd immunity," telling reporters erroneously that New York, Chicago, and New Orleans had already reached herd immunity. Trump told the Republican National Convention in late August, "We are aggressively sheltering those at highest risk, especially the elderly, while allowing lower-risk Americans to safely return to work and to school, and we want to see so many of those great states be open. We want them to be open. They have to be open. They have to get back to work."[91]

Dr. Jeffrey Koplan, CDC director during the Clinton and Bush presidencies, noted: "There comes a time when it makes it very hard to operate effectively, when things are being suggested, requested, ordered that you think are contrary to the containment of the pandemic."[92]

Another former CDC commissioner, Dr. William Foege, wrote a letter to Dr. Redfield on September 23, later made public, asking for Redfield's

[88] Weiland W, Stolberg SG, Goodnough A. Political appointees meddled in C.D.C.'s "holiest of the holy." *The New York Times*. September 12, 2020.

[89] Sun LH, Achenbach J. CDC's credibility is eroded by internal blunders and external attacks as coronavirus vaccine campaigns loom. *The Washington Post*. September 28, 2020.

[90] Sun LH, Achenbach J. CDC's credibility is eroded by internal blunders and external attacks as coronavirus vaccine campaigns loom. *The Washington Post*. September 28, 2020.

[91] Abutaleb Y, Dawsey J. New Trump pandemic adviser pushes controversial "herd immunity" strategy, worrying public health officials. *The Washington Post*. August 31, 2020.

[92] Lipton E, Goodnough A, Shear MD, Twohey M, Mandavilli A, Fink S, Walker M. The C.D.C. waited "its entire existence for this moment." What went wrong? *The New York Times*. June 3, 2020.

resignation, "Silence becomes complicity . . . stand up to a bully. As I have indicated to you before, resigning is a one-day story and you will be replaced, when they fire you, this will be a multiweek story and you can hold your head high."[93]

On April 14, Trump announced that he was halting all funding to the WHO, criticizing its failure to investigate and discipline China for its role in the pandemic. Founded after World War II as part of the United Nations, WHO is the international leader in public health. Its budget comes from participating countries and private foundations, with the United States previously the largest contributor, making up 15% of the WHO budget.[94] Never before had the United States halted its funding to the WHO. Richard Horton, editor of *The Lancet*, was outraged by Trump's decision. "The reality is I believe that President Trump's decision to cut funding to WHO in the middle of a global pandemic constituted a crime against humanity. Is that claim an exaggeration? No, and here is why. WHO exists to protect the health and well-being of the world's people. A crime against humanity is a knowing and inhumane attack against a people."[95]

What Is Our Role in Countering Misinformation?

Most healthcare professionals and scientific publications try to steer clear of politics, not wanting to be viewed as partisan. Times have changed. Dr. Ken Haller, a professor of pediatrics at St Louis University, said, "When you're a doctor, people see you as a doctor no matter what you're doing, they're always asking you questions. What's really just been remarkable to me is how this has really ramped up since we've gotten into this pandemic: Am I safe? Should I believe the C.D.C.?"[96]

---

[93] Stolberg SG. Battered by Trump, the C.D.C.'s director faces pressure to speak out. *The New York Times*. October 10, 2020.

[94] Victor D, Hauser C. What the W.H.O. does, and how U.S. funding cuts could affect it. *The New York Times*. April 15, 2020.

[95] Horton R. *The COVID-19 Catastrophe*. Cambridge, UK: Polity Press, 2020.

[96] Klass, P. How pediatricians are fending off coronavirus myths. *The New York Times*. November 16, 2020.

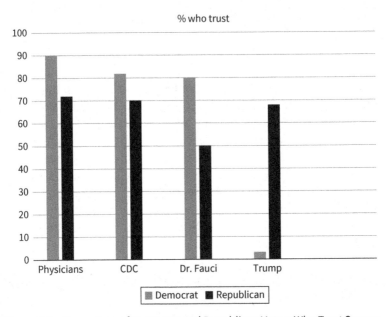

% who trust

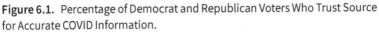

Figure 6.1. Percentage of Democrat and Republican Voters Who Trust Source for Accurate COVID Information.

From: *New York Times*/Sienna College Poll. June 10, 2020.

More than 90% of Americans trust the medical information provided by their healthcare professionals.[97] However, recently party lines have played a major role in public confidence about COVID-19 information. For example, 80% of Democrats but only 50% of Republicans trusted the advice given about the pandemic by Dr. Fauci, whereas 68% of Republicans compared to 3% of Democrats trusted Trump (Figure 6.1).[98]

Healthcare providers have become much more politically outspoken, especially as it applies to social inequity. A *New England Journal of Medicine* article, "written by a Black medical student, a White medical anthropologist, a Black trauma surgeon, and a White clinician educator," suggested that "We believe our health professions, colleagues, societies, and systems need to go

---

[97] National Cancer Institute. HINTS: Health Information National Trends Survey. Accessed Marc 29, 2020. https://hints.cancer.gov/

[98] Sanger-Katz M. On coronavirus, Americans still trust the experts. *The New York Times.* June 27, 2020.

beyond declarations. The health professions must continue to engage with the complex social and structural determinants of health that intersect with politics and law."[99]

The *Scientific American* in its 175-year history had never endorsed a presidential candidate until 2020 when it endorsed Joe Biden. *The New England Journal of Medicine*, never before weighing in on political issues in its 208 years, made this extraordinary rebuke of the Trump administration on October 8, 2020. "The United States came into this crisis with enormous advantages. Along with tremendous manufacturing capacity, we have a biomedical research system that is the envy of the world. We have enormous expertise in public health, health policy, and basic biology and have consistently been able to turn that expertise into new therapies and preventive measures. And much of that national expertise resides in government institutions. Yet our leaders have largely chosen to ignore and even denigrate experts. Anyone else who recklessly squandered lives and money in this way would be suffering legal consequences. Our leaders have largely claimed immunity for their actions. But this election gives us the power to render judgment. Reasonable people will certainly disagree about the many political positions taken by candidates. But truth is neither liberal nor conservative. When it comes to the response to the largest public health crisis of our time, our current political leaders have demonstrated that they are dangerously incompetent. We should not abet them and enable the deaths of thousands more Americans by allowing them to keep their jobs."[100]

[99] Paul Jr DW, Knight KR, Campbell A, Aronson L. Beyond a moment-reckoning with our history and embracing antiracism in medicine. *N Engl J Med*. 2020;83:1404–1406. doi: 10.1056/NEJMp2021812.

[100] The Editors. Dying in a leadership vacuum. *N Engl J Med*. 2020:383:1479–1480.

7

Persistent Medical Problems

During the past year it became increasingly clear that COVID-19 was often not a short-lived medical illness but was leaving its mark on people long after the initial infection. Sorting this out has proven to be one of the most important and poorly understood aspects of the pandemic. I revised the recent clinical classification suggested by the National Institute for Health and Care Excellence (NICE)[1] to categorize patients with persistent symptoms based on the likelihood of organ damage:

1. Severe or moderate COVID with evidence of organ damage/ dysfunction
2. Multiple symptoms lasting longer than 3 months with no evidence of organ damage

Severe or Moderate COVID with Organ Damage/Dysfunction

Cardiac

Hospitalized patients with severe COVID-19 infections often take weeks to months to recover. This is especially common in patients who were in ICUs on mechanical ventilation, as described by Dr. Dhruv Khullar. "They experience weakness, memory loss, anxiety, depression, and hallucinations, and

[1] National Institute for Health and Care Excellence, Royal College of General Practitioners, Healthcare Improvement Scotland SIGN. COVID-19 rapid guideline: Managing the long-term effects of COVID-19. London: National Institute for Health and Care Excellence, 2020. www.nice.org.uk/ guidance/ng188. Accessed Dec 18, 2020.

have difficulty sleeping, walking, and talking. A quarter of them can't push themselves to a seated position; one-third have symptoms of P.T.S.D."[2]

In some patients with severe COVID, there is evidence of ongoing cardiac, pulmonary, and/or neurologic pathophysiologic abnormalities. Myocardial dysfunction in COVID-19 may be related to myocarditis, with or without pericarditis, microvascular disease related to hypoxemia, or stress cardiomyopathy. Twenty-four of 39 elderly patients who died from COVID lung disease had evidence of the virus present in cardiac tissue.[3] None of them had been diagnosed antemortem with myocarditis, but persistent viral infection was associated with increased cardiac inflammation. Dirk Westermann, a cardiologist at the University Heart and Vascular Centre in Hamburg, described these findings, "We see signs of viral replication in those that are heavily infected. We don't know the long-term consequences of the changes in gene expression yet. I know from other diseases that it's obviously not good to have that increased level of inflammation. The question now is how long these changes persist. Are these going to become chronic effects upon the heart or are these—we hope—temporary effects on cardiac function that will gradually improve over time?"[4]

More than three-quarters of 100 unselected patients recovering at home at a mean of 71 days after COVID infection had cardiac abnormalities detected by imaging or elevated high-sensitivity troponin, suggesting persistent myocardial inflammation.[5] These were young patients with a mean age of 49 years and only one-third had been hospitalized with COVID-19. There was no correlation of the cardiac abnormalities with preexisting conditions, cardiac symptoms at the time of initial COVID diagnosis, or severity of the infection. Significant differences were found in cardiac biomarkers and cardiac imaging in these patients compared to healthy controls (Table 7.1). An accompanying editorial said, "Months after a COVID-19 diagnosis, the possibility exists of residual left ventricular dysfunction and

[2] Khullar D. The challenges of post-COVID-19 care. *The New Yorker*. April 23, 2020.

[3] Lindner D, Fitzek A, Brauninger H, et al. Association of cardiac infection with SARS-CoV-2 in confirmed COVID-19 autopsy cases. *JAMA Cardiol*. 2020;5:1281–1285. doi: 10.1001/jamacardio.2020.3551.

[4] Cooney E. Covid-19 infections leave an impact on the heart, raising concerns about lasting damage. *STAT*. July 27, 2020.

[5] Puntmann VO, Carerj ML, Wieters I, et al. Outcomes of cardiovascular magnetic resonance in patients recently recovered from coronavirus disease 2019 (COVID-19). *JAMA Cardiol*. 2020;5(11):1265–1273. doi: 10.1001/jamacardio.2020.3557.

Table 7.1 Cardiac Characteristics of 100 COVID Patients at Average of 71 Days after Recovery Compared to 50 Healthy Controls

Abnormal Results	Number of COVID-19 Patients ($n = 100$)	Number of Healthy Controls ($n = 50$)
Detectable high sensitivity troponin	71	11
Significantly elevated high sensitivity troponin	5	0
Significantly abnormal myocardial native TI image	40	0
Significantly abnormal myocardial native T2 image	22	0
Myocardial late gadolinium enhancement	32	0
Pericardial effusion	22	0

Modified from Puntmann VO, Carerj ML, Wieters I, et al. Outcomes of cardiovascular magnetic resonance in patients recently recovered from coronavirus disease 2019 (COVID-19). *JAMA Cardiol.* July 27, 2020.

ongoing inflammation, both of sufficient concern to represent a nidus for new-onset heart failure and other cardiovascular complications."[6]

A number of echocardiographic studies in COVID patients have revealed right ventricle abnormalities and left ventricular diastolic dysfunction, suggesting inflammatory-induced heart failure with preserved ejection fraction.[7] In a large general population study during the pandemic, there was an increased mortality rate for patients with ST-segment elevation myocardial infarction.[8] Coronary thrombi in patients with ST elevated myocardial infarction during COVID infection demonstrated an excess of neutrophil

[6] Yancy CW, Fonarow GC. Coronavirus disease 2019 (COVID-19) and the heart—Is heart failure the next chapter? *JAMA Cardiol.* 2020;5:1216–1217. doi: 10.1001/jamacardio.2020.3575.

[7] Freaney PM, Shah SJ, Khan SS. COVID-19 and heart failure with preserved ejection fraction. *JAMA.* September 30, 2020. 2020;324(15):1499–1500.

[8] Gluckman TJ, Wilson MA, Chiu S-T, Penny BW, Chepuri VB, Waggoner JW, et al. Case rates, treatment approaches, and outcomes in acute myocardial infarction during the coronavirus disease 2019 pandemic. *JAMA Cardiology.* 2020;5(12):1419–1424. doi: 10.1001/jamacardio.2020.3629.

extracellular traps compared to infarcts in patients who did not have COVID, possibly accounting for the poor prognosis.[9]

There has also been an increase in stress cardiomyopathy (also known as Takotsubo syndrome), with a fourfold rise from pre-pandemic levels in one report.[10] Stress cardiomyopathy usually presents with ST-segment abnormalities, elevated troponin levels, and echocardiogram evidence of myocardial dysfunction in a noncoronary distribution.[11] It was postulated that the psychological, social, and economic stress associated with the COVID pandemic increases the incidence of stress cardiomyopathy in hospitalized COVID patients and may lead to a chronic cardiomyopathy.

COVID-19-associated myocarditis may occur in patients with mild or moderate COVID infection, including in professional athletes, such as Boston Red Sox pitcher Eduardo Rodriguez and Buffalo Bills tight end Tommy Sweeney, both sidelined for the season.[12] Four of 26 athletes from Ohio State University who had mild COVID infections had cardiac MRI findings of myocarditis, although none were symptomatic.[13] Despite these findings, acute or subacute cardiac clinical disease during COVID infections have not been common. For example, one international patient registry of 3,000 hospitalized COVID patients found that only 2% had congestive heart failure, 0.5% had acute coronary syndrome, and 0.1% myocarditis.[14] In a study from London, three-quarters of hospitalized patients had elevated high-sensitivity troponin and slightly abnormal cardiac MRIs, but

[9] Blasco A, Coronado M-J, Hernandez-Terciado F, Martin P, Royuela A, Ramil E, et al. Assessment of neutrophil extracellular traps in coronary thrombus of a case series of patients with COVID-19 and myocardial infarction. *JAMA Cardiol.* December 29, 2020. 2021;6(4):469–474. doi: 10.1001/jamacardio.2020.7308.

[10] Jabri A, Kalra A, Kumar A, Alameh A, Adroja S, Bashir H, et al. Incidence of stress cardiomyopathy during the coronavirus disease 2019 pandemic. *JAMA Network Open.* 2020;3(7):e2014780. doi: 10.1001/jamanetworkopen.2020.14780.

[11] Medina de Chazal H, Del Buono MG, Keyser-Marcus L, et al. Stress cardiomyopathy diagnosis and treatment: JACC state-of-the-art review. *J Am Coll Cardiol.* 2018;72:1955–1971.

[12] Covid-19 is creating a wave of heart disease. Warraich H. *The New York Times.* August 17, 2020.

[13] Rajpal S, Tong MS, Borchers J, Zareba KM, Obarski TP, Simonetti OP, et al. Cardiovascular magnetic resonance findings in competitive athletes recovering from COVID-19 infection. *JAMA Cardiology.* 2021;6(1):116–118. doi: 10.1001/jamacardio.2020.4916.

[14] Linschoten M, Peters S, van Smeden M, Jewbali LS, Schaap J, Siebelink H -M, et al. Cardiac complications in patients hospitalized with COVID-19. *Eur Heart J Acute Cardiovasc Care.* 2020. Nov 21;2048872620974605. doi: 10.1177/2048872620974605.

patients maintained normal systolic function and had no cardiac wall motion abnormalities.[15]

We must await long-term studies to know if congestive heart failure and cardiomyopathy may become an important sequelae of COVID infection. Dr. Marc Pfeffer, a cardiologist at Brigham and Women's Hospital in Boston, worried, "We knew that this virus, SARS-CoV-2, doesn't spare the heart," he said. "We're going to get a lot of people through the acute phase [but] I think there's going to be a long-term price to pay."[16]

Pulmonary

The lungs are the primary target of COVID-19, and an atypical acute respiratory distress syndrome (ARDS) is the presumptive cause of death in most patients. COVID-19 lung disease is characterized by pulmonary vascular dilatation with near normal lung compliance, not seen in typical ARDS.[17] Chest CT reveals ground glass opacities, and the degree of consolidation and fibrosis correlates with mortality. Autopsy studies demonstrate diffuse alveolar damage and microthrombi and macrothrombi, and viral particles have been noted up to 1 month after initial infection.[18] Patients with preexisting pulmonary vascular disease, asthma, and smoking have an increased risk of COVID-associated lung disease. At the time of discharge, 88% of hospitalized, critically ill patients had evidence of persistent lung dysfunction, although 3 months later, following pulmonary rehabilitation, that number had fallen to 56%.[19] Diaphragm muscle weakness has been a contributing factor in COVID-pulmonary pathology and increased expression for ACE-2

[15] Knight DS, et al. COVID-19: Myocardial injury in survivors. *Circulation* Jul 14, 2020. 142(11):1120–1122. doi: 10.1161/CIRCULATIONAHA.120.049252)

[16] Cooney E. "Carnage" in a lab dish shows how the coronavirus may damage the heart. *STAT*. September 4, 2020.

[17] Gattinoni L, Coppola S, Cressoni M, Busana M, Rossi S, Chiumello D. Covid-19 does not lead to a "typical" acute respiratory distress syndrome. *Am J Respir Crit Care Med.* 2020;201:1299–1300.

[18] Borczul AC, Salvatore SP, Seshan SV, Patel SS, Bussel JB, Mostyka M, et al. COVID-19 pulmonary pathology: A multi-institutional autopsy cohort study from Italy and New York. *Mod Pathol* November 2020;33:2156–2168. doi: 10.1038/s41379-020-00661-1.

[19] Zeldovich L. Some signs of recovery from severe Covid lung damage. *The New York Times.* October 18, 2020.

expression and SARS-CoV-2 infiltration correlated with diaphragm fibrosis in a subset of patients who died from COVID-19 infection.[20]

As discussed for cardiovascular complications, there is concern that the COVID-19 pandemic will result in long-range pulmonary complications related to fibrosis and pulmonary vascular dysfunction, with subsequent pulmonary hypertension. In the past, lung transplants were almost never done in patients with pulmonary infections that had irreversibly damaged their lungs but that has changed with COVID-19. As discussed by Dr. Ankit Bharat, the surgeon who performed the first double lung transplant in a COVID patient, "It's such a paradigm change. Lung transplant has not been considered a treatment option for an infectious disease, so people need to get a little bit more of a comfort level with it."[21]

Neurologic

A literature review from January to late July 2020 found a total of 226 cases of ischemic strokes and 35 cases of intracranial bleeding related to COVID.[22] Patient mean age was 64 years. Neuroimaging and autopsy studies suggest that hypercoagulability is the primary cause of these strokes. Although strokes have occurred in less than 5% of hospitalized COVID patients, strokes in young patients have been much more common than expected during the pandemic. For example, from March 23 to April 7, 2020, five COVID-infected patients younger than age 50 presented to a New York hospital system with large-vessel ischemic stroke.[23] In the previous year, in a comparable 2-week span, that hospital saw 0.73 patients <50 years with large-vessel strokes.

---

[20] Shi Z, de Vries HJ, Vlaar APJ, ven der Hoeven J, Boon RA, Heunks LMA, et al. Diaphragm pathology in critically ill patients with COVID-19 and postmortem findings from 3 medical centers. *JAMA Intern Med*. November 16, 2020.

[21] Zeldovich L. Some signs of recovery from severe Covid lung damage. *The New York Times*. October 18, 2020.

[22] Fraiman P, Godeiro Jr C, Moro E, Cavallieri F, Zedde M. COVID-19 and cerebrovascular diseases: A systematic review and perspectives for stroke management. *Front Neurol*. 2020 Nov 5;11:574694. doi: 10.3389/fneur.2020.574694.

[23] Oxley TJ, Mocco J, Majidi S, Kellner CP, Shoirah H, Singh IP, et al. Large-vessel stroke as a presenting feature of Covid-19 in the young. *N Engl J Med*. April 28, 2020. doi: 10.1056/NEJMc2009787

Approximately one-third of COVID-hospitalized patients have central nervous system manifestations, and this is more common in patients with severe infections. In a series of 509 hospitalized patients in Chicago, headaches were present in 38%, encephalopathy in 32%, dizziness in 30%, loss of taste in 16%, and loss of smell in 11%.[24] Risk factors for neurologic complications were severe COVID and younger age. Those with encephalopathy were seven times more likely to die. Only one-third of the patients with altered mental status were able to do normal activities months after discharge. In a study of 222 COVID-19 patients from France with neurologic symptoms, altered mental status was present in 52%, focal central neurologic symptoms in 44%, and peripheral limb weakness in 12%.[25] The neurologic diagnoses were encephalopathy in 30%, stroke in 26%, encephalitis in 10%, and Guillain-Barré in 7%. Severe COVID was present in one-half of these patients.

A UK survey of neurologic and neuropsychiatric complications of COVID-19 in 153 patients found cerebrovascular events in 62%, altered mental status in 31%, and encephalitis in 18%.[26] More than one-half of the patients with altered mental status were classified with a new psychiatric diagnosis, including 10 patients with new-onset psychosis, 6 with a dementia-like syndrome, and 4 with an affective disorder. Fifty percent of the patients with altered mental status were under age 60 years. Dr. Hisam Goueli, a psychiatrist in New York, described his patient with no previous psychiatric symptoms, who months earlier had a mild COVID infection but now was hearing voices telling her to kill her children and herself. "It's a horrifying thing that here's this well-accomplished woman and she's like 'I love my kids, and I don't know why I feel this way that I want to decapitate them. Maybe this is Covid-related, maybe it's not.' Every day, she was getting worse. We tried probably eight different medicines. We don't know what the natural course of this is. Does this eventually go away? Do people get better? How long does that normally take? And are you then more prone to

[24] Liotta LM, Batra A, Clark JR, Shlobin NA, Hoffman SC, Orban SZ, et al. Frequent neurologic manifestations and encephalopathy-associated morbidity in Covid-19 patients. *Ann Clin Trans Neurol.* October 5, 2020;7;11:2221–2230. doi: 10.1002/acn3.51210.

[25] Meppiel E, Peiffer N, Maury A, Bekri I, Delorme C, Desestret V, et al. Neurologic manifestations associated with COVID-19: A multicentre registry. *Clin Microbiol Infect.* November 13, 2020. doi: 10.1016/j.cmi.2020.11.005.

[26] Varatharaj A, Thomas N, Ellul MA, Davies NWS, Pollak TA, Tenorio EL. Neurological and neuropsychiatric complications of COVID-19 in 153 patients: A UK-wide surveillance study. *Lancet Psychiatry.* October 7, 2020. doi: 10.1016/S2215-0366(20)30287-X.

have other psychiatric issues as a result? There are just so many unanswered questions."[27]

ACE2 receptors are present in multiple brain regions, and central nervous system viral invasion has been noted across infected neurons, from the olfactory nerve, via vascular endothelium, or from leukocyte migration across the blood-brain barrier.[28] Although SARS-COV-2 can be recovered from brain tissue, it is likely that the persistent neurologic problems are inflammatory/immune in nature, rather than due to direct viral damage.[29] For example Guillain-Barré syndrome, demyelinating disorders, and myasthenia gravis have each been linked to COVID-19.[30] Cerebrospinal fluid analysis of COVID-19 patients with neurologic disease suggested inflammation but no evidence for viral invasion.[31] Brain post-mortem pathology in patients with neurologic symptoms has revealed reactive gliosis and perivascular inflammation, nonspecific findings seen in many acute critical illnesses.[32] In detailed brain autopsy studies on 18 patients, median age of 50 years and only one with ante-mortem neurologic symptoms, there was no virus detected. Magnetic resonance microscopy revealed punctate hyperintensities in nine patients, corresponding to multifocal microvascular injury in the brain and olfactory bulbs.[33]

[27] Belluck P. Small number of Covid patients develop severe psychotic symptoms. *The New York Times.* December 28, 2020.

[28] Zubair AS, McAlpine LS, Gardin T, Farhadian S, Kuruvilla DE, Spudich S. Neuropathogenesis and neurologic manifestations of the coronaviruses in the age of coronavirus disease 2019. *JAMA Neurology.* May 29, 2020;77(8):1018–1027. doi: 10.1001/jamaneurol.2020.2065.

[29] Mukerji SS, Solomon IH. What can we learn from brain autopsy in COVID-19? *Neurosc Lett.* November 25, 2020. doi: 10.1016/j.neulet.2020.135528.

[30] Fredrich S, Greenberg BM, Hatanpaa KJ. Neurological infections in 2020: COVID-19 takes centre stage. *The Lancet Neurology.* January 2021. https://doi.org/10.1016/S1474-4422(20)30451-8.

[31] Eden A, Kanberg N, Gostner J, Fuchs D, Hagberg L, et al. CSF biomarkers in patients with COVID-19 and neurologic symptoms. *Neurology.* 2021;96:e294–e300. doi: 10.1212/WNL.0000000000010977.

[32] Deigendesch N, Sironi L, Kutza M, Wischnewski S, Fuchs V, Hench J, et al. Correlates of critical illness-related encephalopathy predominate postmortem COVID-19 neuropathology. *Acta Neuropathol.* 2020;140:583–586. doi: 10.1007/s00401-020-02213-y.

[33] Lee M-H, Perl DP, Nair G, Li W, Maric D, Murray H, et al. Microvascular injury in the brains of patients with Covid-19. *N Engl J Med.* December 30, 2020. doi: 10.1056/NEJMc2033369.

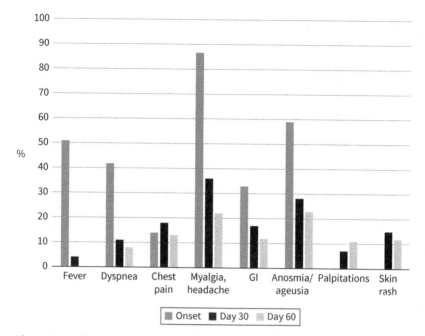

Figure 7.1. COVID-19 Symptoms at Initial Onset, at 30 Days, and at 60 Days.
From: Carvalho-Schneider C, Laurent E, Lemaigned A, Beaufils E, Bourbao-Tournois C, Laribi S, et al. Follow-up of adults with noncritical COVID-19 two months after symptom onset. *Clin Microbiol Infect.* October 5, 2020.

Persistent Organ Dysfunction

In 150 patients from a university hospital in France, two-thirds of patients still were symptomatic at 2 months, including 23% with loss of taste or smell, and 22% with myalgias and headaches. None of these patients had been critically ill. Palpitations and skin rash, not present at onset, were present at 60 days in more than 10% of these patients but no patients were still febrile (Figure 7.1).[34] None of these patients had required ICU admission. Prolonged symptoms were more common in patients age 40–60 years and correlated with more severe initial COVID symptoms, and with an abnormal

---

[34] Carvalho-Schneider C, Laurent E, Lemaigned A, Beaufils E, Bourbao-Tournois C, Laribi S, et al. Follow-up of adults with noncritical COVID-19 two months after symptom onset. *Clin Microbiol Infect.* October 5, 2020. doi: 10.1016/j.cmi.2020.09.052

Table 7.2 Symptoms on Admission and 110 Days Post-Discharge in 120 COVID Patients

Symptoms	On Admission	110 Days Post-Discharge
Dyspnea	73%	42%
Cough	73%	17%
Fatigue	>75%	55%
Cognitive disturbances	6%	34%
Sleep disturbances	ND	31%
Hair loss	ND	20%

Modified from Garrigues E, Janvier P, Kherabi Y, Le Bot A, Hamon A, Gouze H, et al. Post-discharge persistent symptoms and health-related quality of life after hospitalization for COVID-19. *J Infect.* August 25, 2020. doi: 10.1016/j.jinf.2020.08.029.

lung examination. In another report of 120 patients who had been hospitalized with COVID but not critically ill, at a mean of 111 days post-discharge, fatigue was present in 55%, dyspnea in 42%, loss of memory in 34%, and sleep disturbances in 31%.[35] (Table 7.2).

A similar report from Italy found that at 1–2 months after discharge, only 13% of COVID patients were asymptomatic and 55% had three or more symptoms, including 53% with fatigue, 43% with dyspnea, and 2% with musculoskeletal pain.[36,37] In 384 patients discharged from three hospitals in London, at 2 months post-discharge, 70% were fatigued, 53% still reported dyspnea, and 34% persistent cough, although these symptoms were improving.[38] Ninety percent of patients had improved laboratory tests, but

[35] Garrigues E, Janvier P, Kherabi Y, Le Bot A, Hamon A, Gouze H, et al. Post-discharge persistent symptoms and health-related quality of life after hospitalization for COVID-19. *J Infect.* August 25, 2020. 2020 Dec;81(6):e4–e6. doi: 10.1016/j.jinf.2020.08.029
[36] Carli A, Bernabei R, Landi F. Persistent symptoms in patients after acute COVID-19. *JAMA.* August 11, 2020;324;603–605.
[37] Bowles KH, McDonald M, Barron Y, Kennedy E, O'Connor M, Mikkelsen M. Surviving COVID-19 after hospital discharge: Symptom, functional, and adverse outcomes of home health recipients. *Ann Intern Med.* November 24, 2020. doi: 10.7326/M20-5206
[38] Mandal S, Barnett J, Brill SE, Brown JS, Denneny EK, Hare SS, et al. "Long-COVID": A cross-sectional study of persisting symptoms, biomarker and imaging abnormalities following hospitalization for COVID-19. *Thorax.* November 10, 2020. doi: 10.1136/thoraxjnl-2020-215818

30% still had elevated d-dimer levels, and 10% had elevated C-reactive protein. Thirty-eight percent of chest radiographs were still abnormal, including 10% that had worsened.

Loss of smell and taste is of particular interest to follow over time since it is an uncommon symptom in the general population in contrast to headaches, fatigue, and dizziness. In two reports, loss of taste and smell persisted at 2 months in one-third of patients following COVID-19 infection.[39,40] Another study reported a loss of smell or taste in 42% of people who tested positive and 19% of those who had negative COVID-19 tests. These patients were young, mean age 38, and only 5% were hospitalized. At an average of six weeks after a positive test, 26% of these individuals had not recovered their loss of smell.[41] Patients with months of persistent loss of taste and smell described, "I feel discombobulated—like I don't exist. I can't smell my house and feel at home. I can't smell fresh air or grass when I go out. I can't smell the rain. It's also kind of a loneliness in the world. Like a part of me is missing, as I can no longer smell and experience the emotions of everyday basic living."[42] Dr. Sandeep Robert Datta, associate professor of neurobiology at Harvard Medical School, asserted, "You think of it as an aesthetic bonus sense. But when someone is denied their sense of smell, it changes the way they perceive the environment and their place in the environment. People's sense of well-being declines. It can be really jarring and disconcerting. From a public health perspective, this is really important. If you think worldwide about the number of people with Covid, even if only 10% have a more prolonged smell loss, we're talking about potentially millions of people."[43]

[39] Le Bon SD, Pisarski N, Verbeke J, et al. Psychophysical evaluation of chemosensory functions 5 weeks after olfactory loss due to COVID-19: A prospective cohort study on 72 patients. *Eur Arch Otorhinolaryngol.* August 4, 2020.

[40] Carvalho-Schneider C, Laurent E, Lemaignen A, Beaufils E, Bourbao-Tournois C, Laribi S, et al. Follow-up of adults with noncritical COVID-19 two months after symptom onset. *Clin Microbiol Infect.* October 5, 2020. doi: 10.1016/j.cmi.2020.09.052.

[41] Loftus PA, Roland LT, Gurrola II JG, Cheung SW, Chang JL. Temporal profile of olfactory dysfunction in COVID-19. *OTO Open.* December 7, 2020. doi: 10.1177/2473974X20978133.

[42] Rabin RC. Some Covid survivors haunted by loss of smell and taste. *The New York Times.* January 2, 2020.

[43] Rabin RC. Some Covid survivors haunted by loss of smell and taste. *The New York Times.* January 2, 2020.

Multiple Symptoms Lasting Longer Than Three Months with No Evidence of Organ Damage

Approximately 5%–10% of people continue to be symptomatic for longer than 3 months following COVID-19 infection.[44] This includes patients who were never hospitalized but continue to have a variety of perplexing symptoms. These patients have often been labeled as long-COVID syndrome or "long-haulers." My working-case definition of long-COVID includes:

- Prolonged symptoms, more than 3 months after initial infection
- Initial COVID infection usually not severe, not hospitalized
- Multiple symptoms, including fatigue, body aches, headache, dyspnea, cognitive, gastrointestinal, sleep, and mood disturbances
- No evidence of organ damage

Dr. Paul Garner, a UK professor of infectious disease, said, "In mid-March, I developed covid-19. For almost seven weeks I have been through a roller coaster of ill health, extreme emotions, and utter exhaustion. Although not hospitalized, it has been frightening and long. The illness ebbs and flows, but never goes away. The symptoms changed, it was like an advent calendar, every day there was a surprise, something new. A muggy head; acutely painful calf; upset stomach; tinnitus; pins and needles; aching all over; breathlessness; dizziness; arthritis in my hands; weird sensation in the skin with synthetic materials. Gentle exercise or walking made me worse—I would feel absolutely dreadful the next day."[45]

In the largest study of persistent symptoms following COVID infection, 1,700 patients who had been hospitalized in Wuhan China between January 7 and May 29, 2020, were surveyed at a median follow-up time of 186 days.[46] Only 4% of these patients had been treated in an ICU. More than 60%

---

[44] Sudre CH, Murray B, Varsavsky T, Graham MS, Penfold RS, Bowyer RC, et al. Attributes and predictors of Long-Covid: Analysis of COVID cases and their symptoms collected by the Covid symptoms study app. *medRxiv*. doi: https://doi.org/10.1101/2020.10.19.20214494.

[45] Garner P. For 7 weeks I have been through a roller coaster of ill health, extreme emotions, and utter exhaustion. *BMJ Opinion*. May 5, 2020.

[46] Huang C, Huang L, Wang Y, Li X, Ren L, Gu X, et al. 6-month consequences of COVID-19 in patients discharged from hospital: A cohort study. *The Lancet*. January 8 2021. https://doi.org/10.1016/S0140-6736(20)32656-8.

reported fatigue or myalgias, 26% had sleep disturbances, and 23% mood disturbances. More women than men had prolonged symptoms.

The COVID-19 Symptom Study used a mobile application to provide self-reported data from the general population, enrolling more than 2 million participants from the United Kingdom with possible COVID symptoms.[47] Of more than 4,000 cases of probable COVID, 13% had symptoms for >28 days and 5% symptoms lasting longer than 56 days, meeting their criteria for long-COVID. Less than 1% reported a positive COVID PCR test; therefore, it is difficult to extrapolate whether persistent symptoms were related to a true COVID infection in the majority of respondents. In those classified as long-COVID, persistent fatigue and headaches were present in 90% at 28 days and 70%–85% at 56 days (Figure 7.2). Loss of smell was still present in 65% at 56 days. Women, older patients, and those who had multiple symptoms initially were more likely to be categorized as possible long-COVID syndrome. The symptoms in the first week of illness most predictive of long-COVID were fatigue, headache, dyspnea, hoarse voice, and myalgias. Females between age 50–60 years had the highest odds of long-COVID.

Persistent fatigue long after an initial COVID-19 infection has been associated with apathy and cognitive deficits. Chris Long was hospitalized seven times following his initial COVID hospitalization in March 2020, and in December described his exhaustion and cognitive issues, "I read 10 pages in one of my textbooks and then five minutes later, after a phone call, I can't remember what I read."[48] Dr. Vincent Chopra, chief of hospital medicine at the University of Michigan, noted that brain fog is a "clear cognitive issue that is evident when they get readmitted. It is there and real." Dr. Serena Spudich, chief of neurological infections and global neurology at Yale School of Medicine, suggests that inflammatory/immune mechanisms are responsible, "when antibodies mistakenly attack nerve cells."[49] Neurophysiologic tests revealed reduction in post-exertion corticomotor inhibition suggestive of GABAergic dysfunction.[50]

[47] Sudre CH, Murray B, Varsavsky T, Graham MS, Penfold RS, Bowyer RC, et al. Attributes and predictors of Long-Covid: Analysis of COVID cases and their symptoms collected by the Covid symptoms study app. *medRxiv.* https://doi.org/10.1101/2020.10.19.20214494.

[48] Belluck P. He was hospitalized for Covid-19. Then hospitalized again. And again. *The New York Times.* December 30, 2020.

[49] Belluck P. "I feel like I have dementia": Brain fog plagues Covid survivors. *The New York Times.* October 12, 2020.

[50] Ortelli P, Ferrazzoli D, Sebastianelli L, Oliviero A, Kofler M, Versace V. Neuropsychological and neurophysiological correlates of fatigue in post-acute patients with neurological

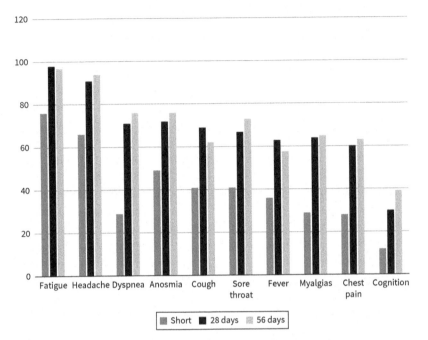

Figure 7.2. Persistent COVID-19 Symptoms from Self-Report COVID-19 Symptom Survey Categorized as Short (Symptoms <10 days) and Long (Symptoms >28 days or >56 days).

From: Sudre CH, Murray B, Varsavsky T, Graham MS, Penfold RS, Bowyer RC, et al. Attributes and predictors of Long-Covid: Analysis of COVID cases and their symptoms collected by the COVID symptoms study app. *medRxiv*. doi: https://doi.org/10.1101/2020.10.19.20214494.

Confusion was documented in only 6% of patients hospitalized with COVID-19 but in 30%–40% 2–3 months following hospital discharge.[51] Lisa Mizelle, a nurse practitioner at an urgent care clinic who had COVID in July, described that when she went back to work 3 months after the initial COVID infection, "I leave the room and I can't remember what the patient just said.

manifestations of COVID-19: Insights into a challenging symptom. *J Neurol Sci*. December 14, 2020. https://doi.org/10.1016/j.jns.2020.117271.

[51] Garrigues E, Janvier P, Kherabi Y, Le Bot A, Hamon A, Gouze H, et al. Post-discharge persistent symptoms and health-related quality of life after hospitalization for COVID-19. *J Infect*. August 25, 2020. doi: 10.1016/j.jinf.2020.08.029

It scares me to think I'm working. I feel like I have dementia."[52] Erica Taylor, a 31-year-old lawyer, described her symptoms months after COVID, "One morning, everything in my brain was white static. I was sitting on the edge of the bed, crying and feeling 'something's wrong, I should be asking for help,' but I couldn't remember who or what I should be asking. I forgot who I was and where I was. I'm scared. I really want to get back to work. But, I keep getting really tired and really confused."[53]

Dr. Anthony Fauci said in July 2020, "Anecdotally, there's no question that there are a considerable number of individuals who have a post-viral syndrome that really, in many respects, can incapacitate them for weeks and weeks following so-called recovery and clearing of the virus, highly suggestive of myalgic encephalomyelitis/chronic fatigue syndrome."[54] In early December 2020, the NIH held a 2-day meeting dedicated to long-COVID syndrome, Dr. Fauci commented that "this is going to be a significant public health issue," and Dr. John Brooks, the chief medical officer of the CDC's Covid response, predicted that "long-COVID would affect on the order of tens of thousands in the United States and possibly hundreds of thousands. If you were to ask me what do we know about this post-acute phase, I really am hard pressed to tell you that we know much. This is what we're really working on epidemiologically to understand what it is, how many people get it, how long does it last, what causes it, who does it affect, and then of course, what can we do to prevent it from happening."[55]

Fauci's comparing post-COVID syndrome to chronic fatigue syndrome (CFS), referred to in the United Kingdom as benign myalgic encephalomyelitis (BME), mirrors my own logic. Much of my career was dedicated to patients with identical symptoms, including chronic fatigue, widespread pain, chest wall pain, palpitations, "brain fog," abdominal pain and diarrhea, numbness and tingling, and mood and sleep disturbances. Depending on the predominate complaints and the clinician's specialty, these patients may be diagnosed with fibromyalgia, CFS/BME, irritable bowel syndrome (IBS), or

---

[52] Belluck P. "I feel like I have dementia": Brain fog plagues Covid survivors. *The New York Times*. October 12, 2020.

[53] Belluck P. "I feel like I have dementia": Brain fog plagues Covid survivors. *The New York Times*. October 12, 2020.

[54] Rubin R. As their numbers grow, COVID-19 "long haulers" stump experts. *JAMA*. 2020;324(14):1381–1383. doi:10.1001/jama.2020.17709.

[55] Belluck P. Covid survivors with long-term symptoms need urgent attention, experts say. *The New York Times*. December 4, 2020.

chronic pelvic/bladder pain syndrome. Applying the following overarching questions about these disorders to post-COVID syndrome is instructive.

Do Persistent, Multiple Symptoms Follow Viral Infections?

Post-viral syndromes, such as following Ross River and Coxiella virus, are not rare. Some patients reported prolonged symptoms following SARS infections, and their symptoms and subsequent sleep studies were similar to those noted in patients with CFS and fibromyalgia.[56] CFS/BME was reported in nurses and other HCWs following widespread community and hospital infections. Viral or bacterial gastroenteritis may trigger IBS and bladder infections trigger chronic pelvic/bladder pain syndrome. Anecdotally, about one-third of fibromyalgia patients report that their symptoms began following a viral infection.

There is no evidence that the virus is directly causing these chronic symptoms. Initial studies suggested that Epstein-Barr was the cause of CFS, but that proved incorrect. Some patients and support groups have objected to the term "post-viral syndrome." As Dr. Paul Garner said, "The least helpful comments were from people who explained to me that I had post-viral fatigue. I knew this was wrong. I spoke to others experiencing weird symptoms, which were often discounted by those around them as anxiety, making them doubt themselves. And too, people report that their families do not believe their ever-changing symptoms, that it is psychological, it is the stress."

Is There Organ Damage?

Despite more than a half-century of intense research, CFS/BME, fibromyalgia, IBS, and related disorders are not associated with organ damage. The absence of organ pathology or abnormal blood and radiologic tests is frustrating to physicians and patients. Now, patients with post-COVID

---

[56] Moldofsky H, Patcai J. Chronic widespread musculoskeletal pain, fatigue, depression and disordered sleep in chronic post-SARS syndrome; A case-controlled study. *BMC Neurol.* May 24, 2011. doi: 10.1186/1471-2377-11-37.

syndrome are experiencing the same frustration, and why patients such as Dr. Garner often feel discounted.

It is essential that every patient with prolonged symptoms following COVID-19 undergo a comprehensive evaluation to exclude organ pathology. This evaluation should focus on the nature of current symptoms and should include lying and standing pulse and blood pressure and a complete general physical examination. Screening tests for persistent systemic inflammation might include CBC; ESR or CRP; d-dimer; ferritin; thyroid, kidney, and liver function tests; and, if respiratory symptoms persist, a chest CT scan. Referral to cardiology, pulmonary, or neurology specialists should be based on symptom severity and prior evaluation. Many individuals meeting the criteria for long-COVID syndrome have no evidence for organ damage after extensive testing.

Sometimes the absence of objective signs of disease leads to the misconception that there is no physiological basis for the chronic symptoms. Absence of organ damage does not imply absence of organ dysfunction. Dr. Jeffrey Siegelman, an emergency medicine physician in Atlanta, described the search for objective markers for his own bout of post-COVID symptoms: "My test results were normal . . . imaging, laboratory results, oxygen saturation were all fine. But I did not feel fine, and still do not. I have had a rotating constellation of symptoms, different each day and worse each evening: fever, headache, dizziness, palpitations, tachycardia, and others. As a result, I have been reminded of the need to listen to the patient first, even in the absence of conclusive testing. The next time I care for someone with vague abdominal pain, or fatigue, or paresthesia, or any of the myriad conditions that are uncomfortable on the inside but look fine on the outside, I will remember that these symptoms are real and impactful for patients. There is a marked difference between tests being within normal limits and a patient being well."[57]

There is incontrovertible evidence for central nervous system (CNS) and autonomic nervous system (ANS) dysfunction in fibromyalgia, CFS/BME, and related disorders. These include abnormalities in functional imaging of the brain or in stress reactivity of the ANS. This generalized CNS and ANS hypersensitivity is thought to promote chronic sleep, mood, and cognitive

---

[57] Siegelman JN. Reflections of a COVID-19 long hauler. *JAMA.* 2020;324(20):2031–2032. doi:10.1001/jama.2020.22130.

disturbances, as well as gastrointestinal and genital-urinary irritability. My suspicion is that similar abnormalities will be noted in long-COVID syndrome. For example, orthostatic intolerance has been common in post-COVID syndrome and, if suspected, patients should be referred for formal autonomic testing.

What Is the Best Therapy?

If the prolonged symptoms interfere with a patient's daily activities, the patient should be referred for multidisciplinary management, with rehabilitation and mental health specialists. Fortunately, a number of US academic medical centers have established such multidisciplinary units to further evaluate patients with long-COVID syndrome. Dr. Ann Parker, who codirects such a clinic at Johns Hopkins Medical Center reported, that "Approximately three months after their acute illness, more than half of our patients have at least a mild cognitive impairment. We're also seeing substantial mental health impairments."[58] It is encouraging that scientists and public health experts are taking long-COVID seriously, as Dr. Tedros Adhanom Ghegreyesus, Director General of WHO, said in October 2020, "We have heard loud and clear that long-COVID needs recognition, guidelines, research and ongoing patient input and narratives, to shape the WHO response from here on."[59] The NICE guidelines from the United Kingdom and WHO have released long-COVID guidelines and the National Health Service has launched 40 long-COVID clinics in the United Kingdom.

Most multidisciplinary programs utilize a biopsychological illness model, refraining from physical or psychological dualism. Too often HCWs and patients assume that a biopsychological illness model downplays the physical nature of symptoms. This has certainly been the experience for many patients with CFS and fibromyalgia, and their frustration led to vocal outcry from various support groups. Dr. Pooja Yerramilli, a resident at Massachusetts General Hospital, was hesitant to call herself a long-hauler because, " . . .long-haulers evoke the same reactions that we have to patients

---

[58] Belluck P. Covid survivors with long-term symptoms need urgent attention, experts say. *The New York Times*. December 4, 2020.
[59] Editorial. Long COVID: Let patients help define long-lasting COVID symptoms. *Nature*. October 7, 2020.

with other medically inexplicable conditions like chronic fatigue syndrome or fibromyalgia. Namely, we assume that their symptoms are psychologically driven, perhaps implicitly by stress and explicitly by secondary gain.... It is difficult to accept long haulers as a group that warrants our attention."[60] However, once Dr. Yerramilli met other patients with identical symptoms, she noted, "They started support groups in which they could discuss their lingering symptoms. Membership in these groups quickly expanded globally.... I share their struggles. Physicians are taught to weigh objective evidence over subjective experience. Instead, perhaps we ought to humbly admit uncertainty and maintain the openness and curiosity required to ask the right questions."[61]

A group of HCWs who were experiencing long-COVID symptoms worried that the NICE guidelines "overly focused on self-management, psychological support, and rehabilitation, resulting in the potential for 'watered-down' versions of NHS long-COVID clinics that do not provide thorough physical assessment of patients. There are implicit assumptions about the nature of long-COVID, which could result in some likening it to post-viral fatigue and may lead to providers over-emphasizing a psychological component. At the very early stage of any new disease, it is unwise to presume parallels with other conditions. This approach risks mismanagement and missed pathology."[62] It is essential that long-term studies, including both hospitalized and nonhospitalized patients, are conducted to better understand the natural history, pathophysiology, and management of long-COVID syndrome.

Mara Gay, a member of the *New York Times*' editorial board and "one of millions of people still fighting to regain their full health months after surviving Covid-19," recounted "the small army of people who are helping me heal. Beating a novel disease in a broken healthcare system means finding the right doctors and asking the right questions. That takes professional skills, time and resources that many people don't have. Many survivors, like me, will need physical therapy, and likely emotional support as well. Though the

---

[60] Yerramilli P. I have all the symptoms of a Covid-19 long-hauler—but I'm hesitant to identify myself as one. *STAT.* October 26, 2020.

[61] Yerramilli P. I have all the symptoms of a Covid-19 long-hauler-but I'm hesitant to identify myself as one. *STAT.* October 26, 2020.

[62] Gorna R, MacDemott N, Rayner C, O'Hara M, Evans S, Agyen L, et al. Long COVID guidelines need to reflect lived experience. *The Lancet.* December 18, 2020. doi: 10.1016/S0140-6736(20)32705-7.

Covid-19 survivor groups that have popped up in recent months have been a good resource for many people, they can also be overwhelming and aren't a substitute for individualized care or dedicated research efforts. I am feeling so much better these days. I am running again, and breathing easier all the time. I am stronger every day, and well on my way to recovery. But I can't do it alone. None of us can."[63]

Mental Health

Almost 50% of the population reported depressive symptoms during the pandemic with triple the rate of moderate to severe depression compared to before the pandemic (Table 7.3).[64] Individuals with lower socioeconomic resources and those with greater COVID-stressors, such as job loss, had greater odds of depression.

A CDC report found a fourfold increase in depression (24% versus 6%) and a threefold increase in anxiety (26% versus 8%) in the US population during June 2020 compared to June 2019.[65] During the pandemic, 40% of Americans reported adverse mental health or behavioral health disorders, including 31% with depression/anxiety, 26% with PTSD symptoms, and 13% who either began or increased substance abuse.[66] Younger adults, racial/ethnic minorities, essential workers, and unpaid adult caregivers had the highest risk of poor mental health outcomes, increased substance use, and risk of suicidal ideation. Twice as many adults had suicidal ideation during the pandemic compared to the previous year, including 25% of survey respondents age 18–24 who had seriously considered suicide during the previous 30 days. Maria Oquendo professor of psychiatry at the University of Pennsylvania, commented, "It's understandable given what's happening. It would be strange if you didn't feel anxious and depressed. This virus is not

[63] Gay M. What it takes to heal; from Covid-19. *The New York Times.* December 31, 2020.

[64] Ettman CK, Abdalla SM, Cohen GH, Sampson L, Vivier PM, Galea S. Prevalence of depression symptoms in US adults before and during the COVID-19 pandemic. *JAMA Network Open.* 2020;3(9):e2019686. doi:10.1001/jamanetworkopen.2020.19686.

[65] CDC. National Center for Health Statistics. Early release of selected mental health estimates based on data from the January–June 2019 National Health Interview Survey. Atlanta, GA: US Department of Health and Human Services, CDC, National Center for Health Statistics; 2020. https://www.cdc.gov/nchs/data/nhis/earlyrelease/ERmentalhealth.

[66] Czeisler ME, Lane RI, Petrosky E, Wiley JF, Christensen A, Njal R, et al. Mental health, substance use, and suicidal ideation during the covid-19 pandemic—United States, June 24–30, 2020. *MMWR.* August 14, 2020. 2020;69(32):1049–1057.

Table 7.3 Prevalence of Depression Symptoms in US Adults before and during the Pandemic

Depression Symptoms	% Before COVID-19	% During COVID-19
None	75	48
Mild	16	25
Moderate	6	15
Moderately Severe	2	8
Severe	0.7	5

Modified from Ettman, et al. *JAMA Network Open.* 2020;3(9):e2019686.

like a hurricane or earthquake or even terrorist attack. It's not something you can see or touch, and yet the fear of it is everywhere."

After just 1 month of the pandemic in the United Kingdom, there was a significant increase in mental distress in the general population.[67] The increased mental distress was most profound in those who had been employed prior to the pandemic, younger individuals, women, and those living with preschool children. Social isolation and quarantine increased stress, fear, and anger, and quarantine duration correlated with adverse mental health. UK researchers recommended methods to mitigate the effects of isolation[68]:

- Keep quarantine as short as possible
- Provide as much information as possible
- Provide adequate supplies
- Reduce boredom and enhance communication
- Rely on voluntary rather than mandatory isolation

As the pandemic surged on, mental health issues worsened. Preexisting mental and physical disease, daily hours of COVID-19-related media

[67] Pierce M, Hope H, Ford T, Hatch S, Hotopf M, John A, et al. Mental health before and during the COVID-19 pandemic: A longitudinal probability sample survey of the UK population. *Lancet Psychiatry.* October 2020;7:883–892. doi: 10.1016/S2215-0366(20)30308-4.

[68] Brooks SK, Webster RK, Smith LE, Woodland L, Wessely S, Greenberg N, et al. The psychological impact of quarantine and how to reduce it: rapid review of the evidence. *Lancet.* March 14–20, 2020. doi: 10.1016/S0140-6736(20)30460-8.

exposure, exposure to conflicting COVID-19 information in media, and work/financial stress were all associated with psychological distress and depressive symptoms.[69,70] Dr. Erin Marcus, a professor of clinical medicine at the University of Miami, said, "Along with the resurgence of covid-19, an insidious and less perceptible pandemic has arisen: one of anxiety, depression, and grief. It's a phenomenon I've seen among people seeking help in the primary care clinic where I work. I think of the woman who, after her mother and sister died of covid, lost the motivation to take her diabetes medication, or do much of anything else. The man who recovered from covid but who now can't sleep because of flashbacks to his time in the hospital. The woman whose adult children recovered from covid—but who is so anxious about venturing out of her tiny apartment that her normally well-controlled blood pressure has rocketed to dangerously high levels."[71]

Massive mental health budget cuts with shortages of psychiatric beds and mental health professionals existed in the United States long before the pandemic. In 2018–2019 about 50% of Americans said they wished to seek mental healthcare for themselves or family members but three-quarters of those reported limited options, because of high cost and poor insurance coverage.[72] Insurance companies have consistently denied or limited mental health coverage despite the fact that 75% of Americans believe that mental health is just as important as physical health.[73] Before the pandemic, the United States was losing $1 trillion in economic productivity yearly from depression and anxiety, yet it was estimated that every dollar spent on evidence-based care for depression and anxiety returns 5 dollars.[74]

[69] Holman EA, Thompson RR, Garfin DR, Silver RC. The unfolding COVID-19 pandemic: A probability based, nationally representative study of mental health in the U.S. *Sciences Advances.* September 23, 2020. doi: 10.1126/sciadv.abd5390.

[70] Carey B. Tsunami or ripple? The pandemic's mental toll is an open question. *The New York Times.* June 21, 2020.

[71] Marcus EN. Covid-19 has shed light on another pandemic of depression, anxiety and grief. *The Washington Post.* November 24, 2020.

[72] Wood P, Burwell J, Rawlett K. New study reveals lack of access as root cause for mental health crisis in America. National Council for Behavioral Health. October 10, 2018. Thenationalcouncil.org. Accessed December 16, 2020.

[73] Wood P, Burwell J, Rawlett K. New study reveals lack of access as root cause for mental health crisis in America. National Council for Behavioral Health. October 10, 2018. Thenationalcouncil.org. Accessed December 16, 2020.

[74] Brunier A, Drysdale C. COVID-19 disrupting mental health services in most countries, WHO survey. WHO. October 5, 2020.

According to the WHO, more than 90% of countries reported an increased demand for mental health services during the pandemic, but the average country was spending only 2% of their annual health budget on mental health.[75] During COVID, Massachusetts lost 300 pediatric and adult psychiatric beds.[76] Steve Winn, CEO of a behavioral health network in Massachusetts, fretted, "It was hard to find a bed before Covid-19. Shipping young people hours away from their family to a hospital bed in another part of the state right now can be difficult."[77]

Sleep disturbances, which correlate with increases in mood disorders, also skyrocketed during the pandemic. In Italy, 57% of the general population reported sleep disturbances during the pandemic.[78] Dr. Alon Avidan, a neurologist who directs the UCLA Sleep Disorders Center, noted, "With covid-19, we recognize that there is now an epidemic of sleep problems. Patients who used to have insomnia, patients who used to have difficulty falling asleep because of anxiety, are having more problems. Patients who were having nightmares have more nightmares."[79]

Even before the pandemic, 40% of college students described themselves as "so depressed that it was difficult to function."[80] During the pandemic, depression and suicide ideation worsened in young adults, exacerbated by increased isolation and loneliness. In September 2020, one-half of youth age 11–17 reported self-harm or suicidal thoughts, and only 27% had received treatment for depression.[81]

Younger children also suffered increased mental health issues during the pandemic, including a fourfold increase in emergency visits for a psychiatric crisis.[82] A WHO survey of 130 countries published in October 2020

[75] Brunier A, Drysdale C. COVID-19 disrupting mental health services in most countries, WHO survey. WHO. October 5, 2020.

[76] Rapoport R. "Every day is an emergency": The pandemic is worsening psychiatric bed shortages nationwide. *STAT*. December 25, 2020.

[77] Rapoport R. "Every day is an emergency": The pandemic is worsening psychiatric bed shortages nationwide. *STAT*. December 25, 2020.

[78] Partinen M. Sleep research in 2020. COVID-19 related sleep disorders. *The Lancet Neurology*. January 1, 2021. 2021;20(1):15–17. https://doi.org/10.1016/S1474-4422(20)30456-7.

[79] Brulliard K, Wan W. The pandemic is ruining our sleep. Experts say "coronasomnia" could imperil public health. *The Washington Post*. September 3, 2020.

[80] American College Health Association. National College Health Assessment. Spring 2019. ACHA.org/documents/ncha/NCJHA-II

[81] Mental Health America. The state of mental health in America. Mhanational.org. Accessed December 16, 2020.

[82] Tanner L. ER visits, long waits climb for kids in mental health crisis. *The Boston Globe*. December 5, 2020.

found that 60% of the countries were experiencing disruptions to mental health services for their children and teens.[83] Elementary and high school students were also hit hard by social isolation during school shutdowns, as expressed by 14-year-old Aya Raji, "I felt like I was trapped in my own little house and everyone was far away. When you're with friends, you're completely distracted and you don't think about the bad stuff going on. During the beginning of quarantine, I was so alone. All the sad things I used to brush off, I realized I couldn't brush them off anymore."[84] The Well Being Trust predicted that the COVID pandemic will result in 70,000 increased "deaths of despair," defined as avoidable deaths from alcohol, drugs, guns, and suicide. "Deaths of despair have been on the rise for the last decade, and in the context of COVID-19, will be seen as an epidemic within the pandemic."[85]

[83] Tanner L. ER visits, long waits climb for kids in mental health crisis. *The Boston Globe.* December 5, 2020.

[84] Goldberg E. Teens in Covid isolation: "I feel like I was suffocating." *The New York Times.* November 12, 2020.

[85] Petterson S, Westfall JM, Miller BF. Projected deaths of despair during COVID-19. Well Being Trust. Robert Graham Center. https://wellbeingtrust.org/areas-of-focus/policy-and-advocacy/reports/projected-deaths-of-despair-during-covid-19/. Accessed January 3, 2021.

8
The Way Forward

We can all see an end to the pandemic with the amazing efficacy of COVID-19 vaccines. Yet it will be months or even years before most of the world's population has been vaccinated. Dr. Daniela Lamas, newly vaccinated, approached the start of 2021 "still on a pendulum swinging between hope and despair. And now, with headlines about the wealthy trying to pay to jump the line, and images of politicians getting vaccinated before many nursing home residents, it is so easy for some to fear that their time will never come. The vaccine selfies tell us to hold on. For the first time in months, I feel time is moving forward again, and I can let myself believe that our current reality is not forever."[1] The ultimate success of the vaccine will be determined in large part by its equitable, global distribution as well as a renewed confidence in public health and scientific guidelines. These are the same issues that have dogged the dismal US pandemic response: weak public health and global health priority, healthcare inequities, notably in minorities and in the elderly, inadequate primary care and mental health resources, poor protection of our healthcare workers, and mistrust of science. Addressing these issues not only is essential to ending this pandemic but also to better protect ourselves for the future.

Public Health Priority

Former US Surgeon General C. Everett Koop said, "Health care is vital to all of us some of the time, but public health is vital to all of us all of the time."[2] Public health emphasizes societal rather than individual health, but

[1] Lamas DJ. I got vaccinated. But the shot won't save my dying patients. *The New York Times*. December 29, 2020.
[2] Gawande A. We can solve the coronavirus-test mess now—if we want to. *The New Yorker*. September 2, 2020.

Americans focus on health as a personal choice. Public health emphasizes disease prevention rather than treatment. Yet our healthcare system is devoted almost exclusively to treatment, with less than 3% of the country's $3.6 trillion total annual healthcare bill spent on public health. Dr. Tom Frieden, former CDC director, said about public health, "It's saved the most lives by far, for the least amount of money. But you'd never guess that based on how little we invest in it. America was a paradox—a beacon of science embedded in a culture increasingly suspicious of scientists. No one is going to vote for you or name a hospital wing after you because you kept them from getting something that they didn't think they were susceptible to in the first place. The people who cure diseases are glorified, not the people who prevent them."[3]

Before COVID-19, experts might have predicted that the United States was better equipped to handle a pandemic than most countries. A survey of the preparedness of 195 countries to face a major health emergency was completed in October of 2019.[4] This report, the Global Health Security Index (GHS), found that no country was fully prepared for a major health emergency, like a pandemic, but the United States had the highest GHS ranking, a score of 83.5 out of 100, with its high-quality laboratories, technology, and reputation of the CDC. Looking more closely at the GHS report provides clues to our poor response to the pandemic. Although the United States had the overall highest GHS ranking, it had one of the lowest scores on public confidence in the government.[5] The United States also had low scores on the ability of its citizens to access healthcare, ranking 175th globally due to its large number of under- or uninsured people.

Since the 1980s the United States has gradually reduced its investment in public health, public institutions, and social safety net programs, and during that time we have fallen behind all wealthy countries in key health indicators despite spending more on health than any country in the world.[6] We currently rank 36th in life expectancy with extreme health disparities among our population. The United States relies on a fragmented healthcare system

[3] Interlandi J. Why we're losing the battle with Covid-19. *The New York Times.* July 14, 2020.

[4] Cameron EE, Nuzzo JB, Bell JA. Global Health Security Index: Building collective action and accountability. Accessed August 10, 2020. https://www.ghsindex.org/wp-content/uploads/2019/10/2019-Global-Health-Security-Index.pdf.

[5] Nuzzo JB, Bell JA, Cameron EE. Suboptimal US response to COVID-19 despite robust capabilities and resources. *JAMA.* Sept 16, 2020. 2020;324(14):1391–1392.

[6] Galea, S. *Well.* New York: Oxford University Press, 2019.

with each state funding and supervising its own public health. Such fragmentation proved deadly during the pandemic.

Dr. Sandro Galea wrote, "As long as the public debate around health remains focused on doctors, treatments, and the choices we make as individuals, our health will continue to suffer and we will continue with the pattern of investment that has made American health worse than that of all its peer countries."[7]

Public health is a government function, but many Americans distrust government oversight. There has always been tension between our individual liberty and our public well-being. Public health in the United States has been reactive, peaking during epidemics or threats such as bioterrorism, and uneven, with inadequate coordination among local, state, and federal authorities. Dr. Anthony Fauci said, "There's this attitude that public health measures are getting in the way of opening up the country. It's exactly the opposite. In a prudent way, the public health measures are the gateway, the vehicle, the pathway to opening the country. That's the point that gets lost in this that's so frustrating."[8] Almost 60,000 public health worker positions, one-quarter of its total workforce, have been eliminated since 2008.[9] There are 3,000 health departments in the United States and less than one-third have a single epidemiologist on staff.[10] During Trump's tenure, the United States increasingly defunded government-led health initiatives. In 2019, the global health security and biodefense pandemic team, part of Obama's National Security Council, was disbanded by Trump, a harbinger that the coronavirus response was to be left to the states rather than the federal government. The triple threat said to best fight the pandemic—nationwide surveillance, testing, and tracing—never surfaced in the United States. Beth Cameron, who led the National Security project, noted, "I just never expected that we would have such a lack of federal leadership, and it's been deliberate. In a national emergency that is a pandemic, spreading between states, federal leadership is essential."[11]

[7] Galea, S. *Well.* New York: Oxford University Press, 2019.

[8] Joseph A. The road ahead: Charting the coronavirus pandemic over the next 12 months—and beyond. *STAT.* September 22, 2020.

[9] Interlandi J. Why we're losing the battle with Covid-19. *The New York Times.* July 14, 2020.

[10] Abbasi J. Taking a closer look at COVID-19, health inequities, and racism. *JAMA.* June 29, 2020. 2020;324(5):427–429.

[11] Achenbach J, Wan W, Brulliard K, Janes C. The crisis that shocked the world: America's response to the coronavirus. *The Washington Post.* July 19, 2020.

US public health databases are antiquated and during the pandemic states were not able to report on key parameters, like coronavirus-test turnaround times, rates of mask wearing, or PPE availability. Accurate data on hospital and ICU capacity were not available until December 2020. Emerging digital data platforms should allow for more precision public health data and link that to patient records. COVID-tracking resource centers, such as those sponsored by Johns Hopkins and the University of Minnesota, *The Atlantic*, *The New York Times*, and *The Washington Post*, provided much needed data throughout the pandemic. The United States must learn from this to better integrate health systems with public health information.

Following the CDC and FDA testing missteps in February 2020, COVID testing never caught up with each pandemic surge. These agencies must assure that all Americans can get tested simply and cheaply with rapid, accurate results during the next year. Testing should include genetic epidemiology, essential to detect mutant viral strains, such as the UK variant that increased transmissibility in December 2020. After 9 months of pandemic testing, the United States had sequenced just 0.4% of its COVID cases, ranking 41 among all countries capable of performing genetic sequencing.[12]

Confidence in public health also flagged badly in the United Kingdom. As noted in *The Lancet*, "The government needs to urgently restore public trust and confidence. It must reinstate daily briefings and be open, honest, and transparent about where we are. It must admit to and learn from mistakes, not overstate its capabilities and achievements, and must treat the public as equal partners, working with communities to develop effective health promotion strategies."[13]

Although the COVID-19 pandemic was a global public health disaster, the United States, United Kingdom, and other countries' nationalistic response was to close our borders, lock down and guard our limited health supplies. Dr. Richard Horton, editor of *The Lancet*, suggested that the pandemic should fortify the goal of global health. "The threat this pandemic posed will emphasize the importance of protecting and strengthening the health of civilizations as well as communities—what one might call our planetary health. A country's political parties and civil service will recruit

---

[12] Dennis B, Mooney C, Kaplan S, Stevens H. Scientists have a powerful tool for controlling the coronavirus: Its own genetic code. *The Washington Post*. October 13, 2020.

[13] Gurdasani D, Bear L, Bogaert D, Burgess RA, Busse R, Cacciola R, et al. The UK needs a sustainable strategy for COVID-19. *The Lancet*. December 5, 2020.

more scientists to their ranks. Science literacy will be a necessary requirement for governing. Citizens will demand stronger health services and public health systems."[14]

Restoring the status of the CDC is essential to combating the ravages of the pandemic and, as Dr. Tom Frieden said, its leaders must be allowed to speak out: "C.D.C. has a big podium. You have to tell people what you know, when you know it. Otherwise, you get a lack of alignment. It's not just the public. When you do those briefings, the public health departments and the doctors also learn."[15] The CDC's budget needs to be invigorated and not subject to political whims. Even during the pandemic, $300 million of the CDC's budget was redirected to a vaccine public relations campaign.[16]

The United States must rejoin and strengthen our ties with the WHO. The WHO pushed hard against the global infodemic and established an Information Network for Epidemics, called EPI-WIN.[17] The United States should lead global efforts to dramatically increase the budget of WHO and to fund the UN COVID-19 Global Humanitarian Response Plan.

Rich countries like the United States have reserved large surpluses of vaccine doses, leaving poor countries in the lurch. If all the vaccine doses committed to the United States are delivered in 2021, we could inoculate all our residents four times over.[18] WHO and nonprofits supported by Bill Gates have secured a billion vaccine doses for 92 poor countries, under the program called Covax. Canada, Australia, the United Kingdom, and the European Union all made early financial pledges to support Covax, but Trump refused. Dr. Bruce Aylward, senior adviser for the WHO's global vaccine initiative, said, "The worst possible outcome is you're offering vaccines to a whole country's population before we're able to offer it to the highest-risk ones in other countries." It has been estimated that there will not be enough

[14] Horton R. *The COVID-19 Catastrophe*. Cambridge, UK: Polity Press. 2020.

[15] Weiland N. "Like a hand grasping": Trump appointees describe the crushing of the C.D.C. *The New York Times*. December 16, 2020.

[16] Weiland N. "Like a hand grasping": Trump appointees describe the crushing of the C.C.C. *The New York Times*. December 16, 2020.

[17] Duffy B, Allington D. Covid conspiracies and confusions: The impact on compliance with the UK's lockdown and the link with social media use. NIHR. The Policy Institute. Kin's College, London. June 18, 2020. https://www.kcl.ac.uk/policy-institute/assets/covid-conspiracies-and-confusions.pdf

[18] Twohey M, Collins K, Thomas K. With first dibs on vaccine, rich countries have "cleared the shelves." *The New York Times*. December 15, 2020.

vaccine globally until 2024, and this does not account for the likelihood that COVID vaccine, like influenza, may require yearly doses.

Collaboration of scientists around the world to develop vaccines in record time demonstrated the power of international research cooperation. We must guard against vaccine nationalism, Dr. Galea said. "The United States has not settled the question of whether it regards health as a value worth upholding as a public good. In our indecision on this point, we are rather unique. When we only care about our own health, we are also likelier to tolerate the injustices that often underlie the structural challenges that create poor health for all. Embracing health as a collective value means embracing the compassion that allows us to see how the suffering of individuals connects with the larger forces that produce health."[19] Ryu and colleagues wrote in *The New England Journal of Medicine*, "We have been forced to think about the needs of the whole population more than ever before and that has drawn attention to these issues and helped us develop the vocabulary to discuss them. It is this population-level lens that will be required to truly transform our health care system."[20]

Healthcare Inequities

The United States spends more money on healthcare than any country in the world, with per capita spending 50% to 200% greater than in other economically developed nations.[21] Nevertheless, the United States ranks twenty-sixth in the world for life expectancy, with higher infant mortality, obesity, and diabetes rates than most other wealthy countries. These health burdens fall largely on our minority populations, reflected by the fact that the United States ranks last on measures of health equity among industrialized nations.[22]

[19]   Galea, S. *Well*. New York: Oxford University Press, 2019.

[20]   Ryu J, Russell K, Shrank W. A flower blooms in the bitter soil of the Covid-19 crisis. *N Engl J Med*. June 24, 2020. doi: 10.1056/CAT.20.0321. https://catalyst.nejm.org/doi/pdf/10.1056/CAT.20.0321

[21]   Schneider EC. Health care as an ongoing policy project. *N Engl J Med*. 2020;383:405–408.

[22]   Evans MK. Health equity—Are we finally on the edge of a new frontier? *N Engl J Med*. September 10, 2020. 2020;383:997–999. doi: 10.1056/NEJMp2005944.

Eighty percent of health outcomes are determined by social, rather that medical, factors.[23] These include employment status, education, housing, diet, and transportation. Life expectancy gaps between the richest and the poorest 1% of Americans exceed 10 years for women and 14 years for men and 80% of the difference in life expectancy between Black and White Americans is based on socioeconomic factors.[24] Dr. Galea noted, "It is a sad truth that black Americans have long had poorer health than white Americans. They have a higher risk of many diseases, including heart disease, diabetes, and stroke. They also live consistently shorter lives than whites (though this gap has narrowed in recent years). These health gaps are neither random nor inevitable. They are a consequence of history."[25] During the pandemic, low-income minority communities suffered from limited access to care, testing, and transportation. Work requirements and multigenerational or unstable housing made it impossible to quarantine. Gains in individual and hospital medical coverage and care with the Affordable Care Act and Medicaid expansion were in jeopardy after the pandemic's financial free-fall.

We are the only country in the world that doesn't consider healthcare a universal right. The United States links healthcare coverage to employment, assuring that we have worked to earn our coverage. Workers without employer coverage, those who are self-employed, unemployed, earn low wages or are disabled struggle or often go uncovered. Twenty-eight million Americans, 8.5% of the population, have no health insurance, and that rate is twice as high in Blacks and Hispanics.[26] Eighteen percent of Hispanics and 10% of Black Americans are uninsured.[27] Inadequate health insurance is responsible for adverse health outcomes and needs to be corrected. The pandemic has reinforced the basic need for universal access to high-quality healthcare for every American. As an example, coverage under the Affordable Care Act reduced racial differences in access to care.[28] Bringing more equity to

[23] Blumenthal, D, Fowler EJ, Abrams M, Collins SR. Covid-19-Implications for the health care system. *N Engl J Med.* 2020 Oct 8;383(15):1483–1488.
[24] Woolf SH, Schoomaker H. Life expectancy and mortality rates in the United States, 1959–2017. *JAMA.* 2019;322:1996–2016.
[25] Galea S. *Well.* New York: Oxford University Press. 2019.
[26] Blumenthal, D, Fowler EJ, Abrams M, Collins SR. Covid-19-Implications for the health care system. *N Engl J Med.* 2020 Oct 8;383(15):1483–1488.
[27] Blumenthal, D, Fowler EJ, Abrams M, Collins SR. Covid-19-Implications for the health care system. *N Engl J Med.* 2020 Oct 8;383(15):1483–1488.
[28] Allen H, Sommers BD. Medicaid expansion and health: assessing the evidence after 5 years. *JAMA.* 2019;322:1253–1254. doi:10.1001/jama.2019.12345.

minorities won't be easy since 60% of White Americans believe that the United States has already made the needed changes to give Black Americans equity, and 50% said that any remaining inequities would disappear if Blacks would only "try harder."[29]

Telemedicine has great potential for lessening healthcare inequities, provided we find a way to bridge the digital divide among racial/ethnic minority, rural, and low-income populations. Dr. Daniel Horn described his frustration with telehealth services for his patients with language and technical barriers at his health center serving poorer patients. "We can't build telehealth systems that exclude the 20 to 30% of our patients who are medically vulnerable. Instead, technology should help address long-standing disparities in access to care: A bus driver in a neighborhood like Chelsea, Massachusetts, or a postal worker in the Bronx should be able to complete a video visit with their doctor during a lunch break instead of taking a day off for what amounts to 20 minutes with a doctor."[30]

After the pandemic, Medicare should continue to reimburse telemedicine visits at the same rate as in-person visits. If it does, private insurers will likely follow. Dr. Ateev Mehrotra, a Harvard health expert, said, "Imagine I'm a primary care practice, I've taken a big financial hit already, and I'm trying to decide: Do I make a big investment in telemedicine or not? It's tough for a clinical practice to not know what you'll get paid in a week or two."[31]

The juxtaposition of the pandemic health inequities and "Black Lives Matter" resulted in a series of publications during 2020–2021 in some of our most prestigious medical journals on the impact of systemic racism on health. Nevertheless, as recently stated in the *NEJM*, "When leading medical journals address structural racism, it is often confined to commentaries and editorials, as though these topics are suitable for discussion but not discovery. Broad agreement is needed—by funders, editors, and reviewers— that racism and inequities in social determinants of health more generally are topics as valid for research as biologic markers (and certainly the two can

[29] Cooper B, Cox D, Lienesch R, Jones RP. Anxiety, nostalgia, and mistrust: Findings from the 2015 American Values Survey. Public Religion Research Institute. Accessed May 1, 2020. https://www.prri.org/research/surveyanxiety-nostalgia-and-mistrust-findings-from-the-2015-american-values-survey.

[30] Horn D. Telemedicine is booming during the pandemic. But it's leaving people behind. *The Washington Post*. July 9, 2020.

[31] Kliff S. This is the health system that Biden inherits from Trump. *The New York Times*. December 16, 2020.

be combined). Our fields have much to regret, and we have much still to offer to right our historical wrongs. Let's not sit on the sidelines."[32]

Female HCWs were faced with difficult decisions regarding work and family balance during the pandemic, on top of a long-standing gender pay gap. Even before the pandemic, the gender pay gap in the United Kingdom was 24% for hospital physicians and 34% for general practitioners.[33] During the pandemic there was a significant decline in women authors on research papers, which may have an adverse impact on their careers.[34]

Healthcare research and funding must be recalibrated to reverse these inequities. Race and ethnicity data should be better recorded and tracked. Community healthcare and outreach programs must be better funded and more widely available. Better access to all healthcare, including digital services, is essential to combat existing inequities. During the pandemic Vanderbilt University Medical Center created a health equity program to prevent, identify, and address pandemic-related inequities.[35] Race and ethnicity data were missing in 20%–30% of health records. Real-time data regarding inequity, widely available with dashboards, were essential to the program's success.

Dr. Michele Evans said, "Now is the time to begin to build pathways to health equity as a long-term goal. We are obliged to acknowledge the lethal consequences of the cracks in our nation's foundational tenets of equality, as Covid-19 exposes the cascading conglomeration of public policies reflecting toleration of underfunding of public health, undermining of equitable healthcare access, and the economic, educational, and judicial marginalization of minorities. In the health policy arena, we can begin by recognizing health care as a human right, so that everyone, regardless of race or socioeconomic status, has a fair and just opportunity to be as healthy as possible."[36]

[32] Bailey ZD, Feldman JM, Bassett MT. How structural racism works—Racist policies as a root cause of U.S. racial health inequities. *N Engl J Med.* 2021;384:768–773. doi: 10.1056/NEJMms2025396

[33] Woodhams C, Dacre J, Parnerkar I, Sharma M. Pay gaps in medicine and the impact of COVID-19 on doctors' careers. *The Lancet.* December 15, 2020.

[34] Editorial. Science during COVID-19: Where do we go from here? *The Lancet.* December 19, 2020.

[35] Wilkins CH, Friedman EC, Churchwell AL, Slayton JM, Jones P, Pulley JM, et al. A systems approach to addressing Covid-19 health inequities. *N Engl J Med.* January 2021. NEJM Catalyst 2(1). doi: https://doi.org/10.1056/CAT.20.0374

[36] Evans MK. Health Equity—Are we finally on the edge of a new frontier? *N Engl J Med.* September 10, 2020. 383(11):997–999/. doi: 10.1056/NEJMp2005944

Long-Term Care Facilities and the Elderly

We must pay more attention to healthy aging and improve the long-term care of the elderly. A *Lancet* editorial said, "Long-term care must value the heritage, experience, and contribution of older people, and see them as individuals who are part of a wider social network. The dehumanizing way that COVID-19 has been managed in people in care homes makes a mockery of the purpose of medicine to extend life and allow people to live life in the fullest sense. The long-term care system in many countries is broken and must be reimagined."[37]

Addressing the overwhelming loss of life in residents and workers of long-term care facilities (LTCFs) requires short and long-term changes. The quality of LTCFs should be immediately upgraded and maintained by adequate state and federal oversight. The total restriction of family visitation at LTCFs increased social isolation of seniors and must be rethought. A number of states are loosening their LTCF visiting restrictions and with appropriate testing and PPE availability, family contact can be reestablished.

Facility-wide COVID-19 testing was delayed until May 2020, but we know that universal testing in LTCFs is the only effective means to detect asymptomatic and presymptomatic infections.[38] Preventive, rather than responsive (testing only after a known infection) testing, with attention to genetic viral sequencing, should be routine in LTCFs.[39] Genetic sequencing at LTCFs demonstrated that viral genomes were clustered by facility, suggesting facility-based transmission among residents and staff.[40]

Most importantly, adequate and well-trained staff are essential to stop the tragic impact of COVID-19 on these facilities. There is an immediate need for 150,000 new LTCF workers in the United States and their jobs must be

---

[37] Editors. Reimagining long-term care. *The Lancet*. October 24, 2020.

[38] Sanchez GV, Biedron C, Fink LR, Hatfield KM, Polistico JM, Meyer MP, et al. Initial and repeated point prevalence surveys to inform SARS-CoV-2 infection prevention in 26 skilled nursing facilities—Detroit, Michigan, March–May 2020. *MMWR*. 2020;69:882–886. doi: 10.15585/mmwr.mm6927e1.

[39] Telford CT, Onwubiko U, Holland DP, Turner K, Smith S, Yoon J, et al. Preventing COVID-19 outbreaks in long-term care facilities through preemptive testing of residents and staff members—Fulton County, Georgia, March–May 2020. *MMWR*. September 18 2020;69(37):1296–1299. doi: 10.15585/mmwr.mm6937a4.

[40] Taylor J, Carter RJ, Lehnertz N, Kazazian L, Sullivan M, Wang X, et al. Serial testing for SARS-CoV-2 and virus whole genome sequencing inform infection risk at two skilled nursing facilities with COVID-19 outbreaks—Minnesota, April–June 2020. *MMWR*. September 18, 2020. 2020;69(37):1288–1295. doi: 10.15585/mmwr.mm6937a3.

upgraded from their current poor-wage, high turnover status.[41] A living wage, $20 or more per hour, is needed, and staffing should include a minimum of one RN per shift with at least 4 hours of daily nursing care per resident. The $264 billion paid to LTCFs yearly by Medicaid and Medicare must be accountable to ensure that it goes to healthcare, rather than to profits.[42]

Over time, we must totally reimagine how we care for the elderly. The model of LTCFs where residents share rooms and bathrooms promoted viral transmission. Private rooms are currently used in less than 300 of the nation's 15,000 LTCFs but those with private rooms had much less COVID-19 infections.[43] Dr. Atul Gawande wrote, " . . . most consider modern old age homes frightening, desolate, even odious places to spend the last phase of one's life. We need and desire something more. We end up with institutions that address any number of societal goals—from freeing up hospital beds to taking burdens off families' hands to coping with poverty among the elderly—but never the goal that matters to the people who reside in them: how to make life worth living when we're weak and frail and can't fend for ourselves anymore."[44]

Dr. Louise Aronson explored our inadequate focus on age and disease. "The outsized impact of Covid-19 on elders has laid bare medicine's outdated, frequently ineffective or injurious approach to the care of patients who are the planet's fastest-growing age group and the generations most often requiring healthcare. This unprecedented crisis is exactly why we need to think now about how best to manage the care of sick elders—for their sake and in consideration of near- and longer-term costs and stresses to the healthcare system. Basic standards of health equity demand protocols with elder-specific diagnostic, treatment, and outcome-prediction tools, addressing lower baseline and illness-related body temperatures, atypical disease presentations, and care options geared to the life stage, health status, and life expectancy of older patients."[45] In a study of more than 5,000 COVID

[41] Beilenson P. How a Covid-19 outbreak among staff and residents at an assisted living facility was controlled. *N Engl J Med*. June 30, 2020.

[42] Kim ET. This is why nursing homes failed so badly. *The New York Times*. December 31, 2020.

[43] Span P. How to improve and protect nursing homes from outbreaks. *The New York Times*. May 22, 2020.

[44] Gawande, A. *Being Mortal: Medicine and What Matters in the End*. New York: Henry Holt and Co., 2014.

[45] Aronson L. Age, complexity and crisis—A prescription for progress in pandemic. *N Engl J Med*. April 7, 2020. 2020;383:4–6.

infections in residents of LTCFs, fever, hypoxia, and tachypnea were much less common than in comparison to hospitalized patients of similar age from the community.[46]

The end-of-life horror stories so rampant during the pandemic reinforced the importance of frank and open discussions around talking about death. Only 30% of US adults have completed an advanced healthcare directive and Dr. Jessica Nutik Zitter, a palliative care and critical care doctor in California, said, "Without Covid-19 breathing down our backs, most of us look the other way from death. Even those of advanced age or with serious illness. Having a plan in place, one that doesn't sugarcoat reality, is the best preparation for ensuring that you are treated as you would wish. It also provides needed clarity to your loved ones, as we all navigate this pandemic together."[47] Telehealth was utilized to establish an electronic medical order system for advance care planning during the pandemic.[48] This system, termed eMOLST (Electronic Medical Orders for Life Sustaining Treatment), at Mount Sinai Hospital in New York, was established after many patients at greatest risk for poor COVID-related outcomes were arriving at the emergency department with no information about their advanced care wishes. The investigators recommended that "We encourage our colleagues to recognize that this crisis creates an opportunity to reframe advanced care planning and document care preferences using eMOLST or similar tools in other states."[49]

Putting residents of LTCFs and older people first in line to receive the vaccine was essential, but vaccine hesitancy and availability quickly became an issue in these vulnerable groups. There has been more worry about adverse side effects as Mahine Ebrani, a 79-year-old Queens, New York, LTNF resident, said. "I think if I get the corona shot, I will get the corona."[50]

---

[46] Panagiotou OA, Kosar CM, White EM, Bantis LE, Yang X, Santostefano CM, et al. Risk factors associated with all-cause mortality in nursing home residents with COVID-19. *JAMA Intern Med.* January 4, 2021;181(4):439–448. doi: 10.1001/jamainternmed.2020.7968.

[47] Dr. Jessica Nutik Zitter. Covid or no Covid, it's important to plan. *The New York Times.* April 16, 2020.

[48] Baharlou S, Orem K, Kelley AS, Aldridge MD, Popp B. Rapid implementation of eMOLST order completion and electronic registry to facilitate advance care planning: MOLST documentation using telehealth in the Covid-19 pandemic. *N Engl J Med.* November 3, 2020. https://catalyst.nejm.org/doi/full/10.1056/CAT.20.0385

[49] Baharlou S, Orem K, Kelley AS, Aldridge MD, Popp B. Rapid implementation of eMOLST order completion and electronic registry to facilitate advance care planning: MOLST documentation using telehealth in the Covid-19 pandemic. *N Engl J Med.* November 3, 2020. https://catalyst.nejm.org/doi/full/10.1056/CAT.20.0385

[50] Mandavilli A. The next vaccine challenge: Reassuring older Americans. *The New York Times.* December 14, 2020.

Homebound elders or those in subsidized housing are less likely to line up at the local pharmacy, so coordinated efforts to get them vaccinated will be important. Keeping aging in mind is also critical to vaccine utilization, as discussed by Koff and Williams, from the Human Vaccines Project. "Numerous studies have shown that vaccine efficacy decreases significantly with age, a reduction that is thought to be driven by the progressive age-related decline of innate and adaptive immune responses. If investigators study cohorts of elderly people longitudinally and globally and probe their immune systems with licensed vaccines to distinguish people with effective responses from those without, and apply cutting-edge tools from systems biology and AI, it should be feasible to identify biomarkers for effective immunity in this population, which could then be applied to other vulnerable populations, such as those living in low- and middle-income countries."[51]

Primary Care and Value-Based Care

Primary care in the United States, including family practice, internal medicine, and pediatrics, is undervalued and underpaid. On average, the United States spends 5%–7% on primary care as a percentage of its total healthcare spending (Figure 8.1).[52] This hasn't changed significantly in the past 10 years. In most countries with universal health coverage, like the United Kingdom, primary care is the center of the healthcare setting and 90% of all NHS contacts take place within primary care.[53] Increased investment in primary care is associated with lower healthcare costs and improved population health and continuity of primary care has been associated with decrease in patient mortality.[54] US states with higher ratios of primary-care physicians have lower rates of general mortality, infant mortality, and mortality from specific conditions such as heart disease and stroke.[55] A 10% increase of primary care

---

[51] Koff WC, Williams MA. Perspective: Covid-19 and immunity in aging populations—A new research agenda. *N Engl J Med*. 2020;383:804–805. doi: 10.1056/NEJMp2006761.

[52] Martin S, Phillips Jr RL, Petterson S, Levin Z, Bazemore AW. Primary care spending in the United States, 2002–2016. *JAMA Intern Med*. 2020;180:1019–1020.

[53] Editors. Transforming primary care. *Lancet*. April 30, 2016.

[54] Baker R, Freeman G, Haggerty JL, et al. Primary medical care continuity and patient mortality: A systematic review. *Br J Gen Pract*. 2020;70(698):e600–e611. doi org/10.3399/bjgp20X712289.

[55] Gawande A. The heroism of incremental care. *The New Yorker*. January 23, 2020.

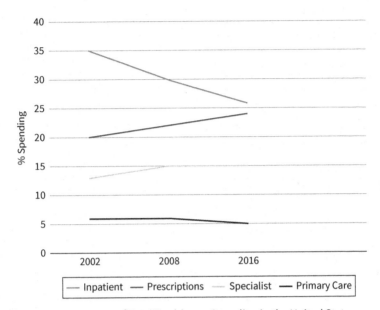

Figure 8.1. Percentage of Total Healthcare Spending in the United States, 2002–2016.

From: Martin S, Phillips Jr RL, Petterson S, Levin Z, Bazemore AW. Primary care spending in the United States, 2002–2016. *JAMA Intern Med.* 2020;180:1019–1020.

coverage in deprived areas of the United Kingdom improved health equivalent to adding 10 years to everyone's life.[56]

Primary-care doctors in the United States have been the most poorly compensated physicians in the United States, confounded by reimbursement that favors specialized procedures over ongoing and preventative care. This has contributed mightily to the current shortage of 14,000 PCPs in the United States [57] Less than one-quarter of graduating medical students are expected to practice primary care, often because of the financial shortfall.[58]

[56] Gawande A. The heroism of incremental care. *The New Yorker.* January 23, 2020.

[57] Marks C. America's looming primary-care crisis. *The New Yorker.* July 25, 2020.

[58] Jackson A, Baron RB, Jaeger J, Liebow M, Plews-Ogan, M, Schwartz MD. Addressing the nation's physician workforce needs. *J Gen Intern Med.* 2014;29:1546–1551. doi: 10.1007/s11606-014-2847-4

The US fee-for-service reimbursement rewards physicians for providing more services, without necessarily greater patient value. The pandemic has renewed an enthusiasm for healthcare reimbursement based on patient value rather than on patient visits. In the United States fee-for-service reimbursement currently accounts for 75% of national payments, whereas value-based reimbursement accounts for just 25%. Dr. Atul Gawande summed it up, "We pay doctors for quantity, not quality . . . we also pay them as individuals, rather than as members of a team working together for their patients. Both practices have made for serious problems."[59] The fiscal disparities between primary and specialty care in the United States are heightened by high rates of reimbursement for technical or specialized procedures but low rates for chronic-disease management, vaccinations, or counseling.

Fixed payment, such as capitation, would provide the financial security sorely needed to shore up United States PCPs. During the pandemic, greater flexibility for reimbursement to PCPs was made available in many states. Maryland, with a primary care program jointly managed by the state and Medicare, kept most PCPs practices open during the pandemic. In Oregon, a state law directs a minimum portion of health insurer expenses to PCPs, with per person payments.

The increased use of telemedicine, remote patient monitoring, and outreach programs during the pandemic are examples of value-based care likely to continue. Preventative, team-based care provides the best value. Home-based and community care will keep patients out of emergency rooms and decrease hospitalizations. The rapid adoption of telemedicine during the pandemic has promoted innovation and flexibility for PCPs. Patients should be enrolled in hospital EHR portals for optimal efficacy and equity of virtual visits.

The pandemic-related decline in medical utilization may provide more clarity on unnecessary medical care, as noted by Dr. H. Gilbert Welch, senior investigator at the Center for Surgery and Public Health. "We are in the midst of an unprecedented natural experiment that gives us an opportunity to determine the effect of a substantial decline in medical care utilization."[60] Before the pandemic an estimated 50 million Americans were subject to healthcare overuse each year at a cost of $106 billion. This

[59] Gawande A. The cost conundrum. *The New Yorker.* May 25, 2009.
[60] Kolata G. Amid pandemic, scientists reassess routine medical care. *The New York Times.* December 12, 2020.

includes 42% of Medicare beneficiaries.[61] It has been increasingly recognized that the routine annual examination has questionable clinical value and PCP's limited time would be better spent on illness prevention. Ten percent of all PCP visits are for an annual physical examination, a cost of $10 billion yearly, and there is little evidence that annual physicals reduce morbidity or mortality.[62] Dr. Horn and colleagues in Boston set up a registry, integrated into electronic health records, that tracks completion of all recommended preventative services.[63] An annual "prevention kit" provides tests that can be done at home, such as fecal immunochemical test, lipid and glycated hemoglobin levels, followed by a virtual healthcare provider visit. Community-based patient navigators help offset any inequities in adequate preventative care.

The United States needs to make a much more substantial investment in mental health/primary care integration. It is estimated that 20% of the US population requires mental healthcare, but more than one-half lack access to that care.[64] Community health centers, currently taking care of 10% of the US population, must be expanded with community and mental health workers as part of PCPs. Stepped care, initiating therapy with the least resource-heavy treatment, should include community organizations, such as support groups and residential and mobile crisis units. Telemedicine mental health coverage must be continued and expanded. During the pandemic, the United States spent trillions of dollars on emergency funding, almost none of which went to mental health. Clinical and research programs in suicide prevention and substance abuse will reduce access to lethal means, including gun control, alcohol, and drugs. Mental health must be recognized as playing an essential role in recovering from this pandemic and in assuring optimal global health in the future.

[61] Oakes AH, Segal JB. The COVID-19 pandemic can help us understand low-value health care. *HealthAffairs*. October 27, 2020.

[62] Mehrotra A, Prochazka A. Improving value in health care-Against the annual physical. *N Engl J Med*. 2015;373:1485–1487. doi: 10.1056/NEJMp1507485.

[63] Horn DM, Haas JS. Covid-19 and the mandate to redefine preventative care. *N Engl J Med*. 2020;383:1505–1507. doi: 10.1056/NEJMp2018749.

[64] Marques L, Bartuska AD, Cohen JN, Youn SJ. Three steps to flatten the mental health need curve amid the COVID-19 pandemic. *Depression & Anxiety*. May 13, 2020.

Healthcare Worker Well-Being

Dr. Suzan Song, a psychiatrist at George Washington University, said, "Physicians take a Hippocratic oath to 'do no harm.' It's time that oath includes doing no harm to ourselves."[65] More than I in 10 adult Americans work in the healthcare field. The pandemic caused enormous strain on the physical and emotional well-being of all HCWs.

Although the vast majority of COVID infections in HCWs were community acquired, adequate PPE has been an ongoing major concern.[66] Lack of PPE for HCWs persisted even late in the pandemic. The United States Strategic National Stockpile had more than 100 million masks in 2009 but that supply was never replenished. Trump said that PPE was a state responsibility. Both in the United States and the United Kingdom, outsourcing PPE supplies to private companies led to ongoing nepotism and profiteering. In the United States, states and hospitals competed for limited supplies, gouging prices up. The Biden administration needs to rein in control of PPE supplies and use the Defense Production Act to increase domestic manufacturing.

Easy access to free and rapid COVID-19 testing must continue.[67] Open and regular communication with hospital administration has dampened the anxiety of HCWs, as noted at the University of Washington, "Our employees require both emotional and practical assistance during this crisis."[68] A framework for addressing pandemic-related clinician's mental health included basic needs such as housing; transportation; child care; PPE; and peer, hospital leadership, and mental health support.[69] New York-Presbyterian Medical Center expanded and added services for its more than 50,000 employees during the pandemic, and their group and individual support

[65] Song S. As the pandemic rages, demoralization deflates health care workers. *STAT*. December 19, 2020.

[66] Frush K, Lee G, Wald SH, Hawn M, Krna C, Holubar M, et al. Navigating the Covid-19 pandemic by caring for our health care workforce as they care for our patients. *N Engl J Med*. 2021; Catalyst.nejm.org 2(1). https://doi.org/10.1056/CAT.20.0378

[67] Frush K, Lee G, Wald SH, Hawn M, Krna C, Holubar M, et al. Navigating the Covid-19 pandemic by caring for our health care workforce as they care for our patients. *N Engl J Med*. 2021; Catalyst.nejm.org 2(1). https://doi.org/10.1056/CAT.20.0378

[68] Kim CS, Kritek PA, Lynch JB, Cohen S, Staiger TO, Sayre C, et al. All hands on deck: How UW medicine is helping its staff weather a pandemic. *N Engl J Med*. April 24, 2020. Catalyst. nejm.org

[69] Schwartz R, Sinskey JL, Anand U, Margolis RD. Addressing postpandemic clinician mental health. *Ann Intern Med*. August 21, 2020. https://doi.org/10.7326/M20-4199

utilized virtual counseling and symptom tracker tools.[70] Telehealth wellness visits, group discussions with debriefing sessions, as well as resources for meditation, virtual yoga, breathing, and sleep were made available in the NYU-affiliated hospitals.[71] HCWs were assured of full access to mental healthcare without any negative career repercussions.

Another hospital program to alleviate HCW stress and provide psychological support, called "Circle Up," was modeled after brief and inspirational meetings utilized by sports coaches or military leaders.[72] These consisted of brief team huddles with the entire team of clinicians and staff, with focus on peer and leadership support. Key to success was "Leveraging an existing patient-focused team conversation, such as a morning huddle, and adapting it to incorporate interprofessional communication and connection will promote the teamwork and support elements without burdening clinicians and staff with additional meetings."[73] At Northwell Health, a Keeping Our Team Members Safe COVID-19 program was endorsed by the staff and resulted in increased staff retention and salaries.[74] Program elements that were best received included adoption of more flexible telemedicine, investment in childcare, free and convenient COVID testing, and symptom monitoring. These are the type of programs that should become standard in large hospital systems.

There were no effective methods to track HCWs' rate of infections, deaths, or long-term mental health impact during the pandemic. For example, the CDC relies on data collected by local health departments, which did not include occupation and job setting until May 2020.[75] There was no in-depth

[70] Smith S, Woo Baidal J, Wilner PJ, Ienuso J. The heroes and heroines: Supporting the front line in New York City during Covid-19. *N Engl J Med*. July 15, 2020. Catalyst.nejm.org.

[71] Schaye VE, Reich JA, Bosworth BP, Stern DT, Volpicelli F, Shapiro NM, et al. Collaborating across private, public, community, and federal hospital systems: Lessons learned from the Covid-19 pandemic response in NYC. *N Engl J Med*. 2020;1(6). https://doi.org/10.1056/CAT.20.0343.

[72] Rock LK, Rudolph JW, Fey MK, Szyld D, Gardner R, Minehart RD, et al. "Circle Up": Workflow adaptation and psychological support via briefing, debriefing, and peer support. *N Engl J Med*. September 22, 2020. Catalyst.nejm.org.

[73] Rock LK, Rudolph JW, Fey MK, Szyld D, Gardner R, Minehart RD, et al. "Circle Up": Workflow adaptation and psychological support via briefing, debriefing, and peer support. *N Engl J Med*. September 22, 2020. Catalyst.nejm.org.

[74] Dowling MJ, Carrington M, Moscola J, Davidson KW. Covid-19 crisis response: First address the safety and well-being of your team. *N Engl J Med*. December 2, 2020. https://catalyst.nejm.org/doi/full/10.1056/CAT.20.0544

[75] Stephenson J. National Academies report urges improvements for tracking COVID-19's burden on health care workers. *JAMA Network*. December 22, 2020. 2020;1(12):e201576.

analysis of essential HCW information, such as intensity of direct patient contact or PPE utilization. A comprehensive HCW data tracking system is essential to better protect our HCWs.

The pandemic demonstrated the advantage of allowing HCWs greater flexibility to practice across state lines. Nursing shortages were buttressed by traveling nurses, but during the winter surge in 2020, their supply and morale were dwindling, as Terri Newland, a critical care traveling nurse, said, "I think a lot of nurses will end up paying for it with their mental and physical well-being. I'm seeing lots of core staff leaving for travel gigs. And I wonder, are we filling some holes by opening up others?"[76] Alexi Nazem, the CEO of a company that sends physicians and nurses to short-staffed hospitals throughout the United States, said in December 2020, "It's been insane. Orders are coming from everywhere. It's crazier than we've ever seen. It's now impossible to distinguish by job. Hospitals are saying, 'Just come. Who knows what we'll need you for.' If and when we hit the limit depends entirely on our national public-health response. But people should know: there is a hard limit. Every day that something doesn't change, we get closer to it."[77]

Before the pandemic, every state required a state medical license for any doctor treating each patient in that state. During the pandemic, many states allowed HCPs to practice across state lines. In November 2020, the Department of Veterans Affairs released a new rule allowing its clinicians to practice across state lines. A more universal acceptance of similar measures would alleviate HCW shortages in underserved regions. In the past, such flexibility was blocked by regulatory concerns, but such concerns have never been substantiated. Flexibility for practicing virtually or in-person across state lines will free up HCWs in the future. Importantly, the nation's shortage of HCWs during the pandemic calls for systematic changes in their fee schedules, career opportunities, and geographic distribution. It was essential that HCWs were the first to receive the COVID vaccine. As WHO Director Tedros Ghebreyesus said, "No country, hospital, or clinic can keep its patients safe unless it keeps its health workers safe."[78]

[76] Khullar D. America is running out of nurses. *The New Yorker*. December 15, 2020.
[77] Khullar D. America is running out of nurses. *The New Yorker*. December 15, 2020.
[78] Editorial. Caring for people who care: Supporting health workers during the COVID-19 pandemic. *The Lancet*. EClinicalMedicine. 2020;28. https://doi.org/10.1016/j.eclinm.2020.100667.

Science and Truth

Vaccine fears persist despite decades of science demonstrating that such worries are unfounded. As the vaccines were approved, coronavirus and vaccine disinformation citations on social media, cable television, and print and online news sites increased, with more than 46,000 mentions on December 3, 2020.[79] One-half of people who were vaccine hesitant said that the risks of COVID-19 were being exaggerated, 37% didn't trust vaccines, 35% didn't trust our healthcare system, and 27% believed that they might get COVID-19 from the vaccine itself.[80] Factors associated with greater vaccine hesitancy have included younger age, Black race, and lower educational levels.[81] Despite the high vaccine efficacy in Phase 3 trials, in December 2020, only 56% of Americans said they were likely to get the vaccine, including only 39% of Blacks (Table 8.1).[82]

Social media can be our ally for providing accurate public health messages and dismantling disinformation. Public health organizations should work with digital platforms to constantly address false information. As healthcare professionals, we must be more vocal.

Jevin West, a data scientist at the University of Washington, has said, "I think scientists need to get out there on the front line, if they are comfortable doing so. By countering misinformation about COVID-19, they can help policymakers avoid introducing harmful policies, improve public understanding of the pandemic and, most importantly, save lives."[83] West founded the University of Washington's new Center for an Informed Public, describing the task to wean out misinformation, "all-consuming, a bit like trying to build a boat while you're floating along in the sea. We should encourage, not discourage, scientists to 'step outside their lane,' especially during a worldwide crisis. As long as they are transparent about their expertise, there is

---

[79] Alba D, Frenkel S. Misinformation peddlers shift gears. *The New York Times*. December 16, 2020.

[80] Silverman E. STAT-Harris Poll: Most Americans won't get a Covid-19 vaccine unless it cuts risk by half. *STAT*. November 10, 2020.

[81] Fisher KA, Bloomstone SJ, et al. Attitudes toward a potential SARS-CoV-2 vaccine: A survey of U.S. adults. *Ann Intern Med*. September 5, 2020. doi:10.7326/M20-3569.

[82] Szilagyi PG, Thomas K, Shah MD, Vizueta N, Cui Y, Vangala S, et al. National trends in the US public's likelihood of getting a COVID-19 vaccine–April 1 to December 8, 2020. *JAMA*. 2021;325(4):396–398. doi:10.1001/jama.2020.26419

[83] Fleming N. Coronavirus misinformation, and how scientists can help to fight it. *Nature*. June 17, 2020. https://www.nature.com/articles/d41586-020-01834-3

Table 8.1. Percent of Adults Likely to Get COVID-19 Vaccine (December 2020)

Demographic	% Likely to Get COVID-Vaccine
White	59
Black	39
Men	62
Women	51
Bachelor's degree or higher	85
OVERALL	56

Modified from: Szilagyi PG, Thomas K, Shah MD, Vizueta N, Cui Y, Vangala S, et al. National trends in the US public's likelihood of getting a COVID-19 vaccine—April 1 to December 8, 2020. *JAMA*. December 29, 2020.

much to gain from more scientists thinking about the problem with their different methodological perspectives and experience . . . lives and trust in science are at stake and we need to do something about it."[84]

Speaking out against the tide of COVID misinformation has not been easy. Dr. Cleavon Gilman, an emergency room physician in Yuma, Arizona, said on December 21, "After you treat patients, intubate them, see people watch their loved ones die, you get to drive home, past the gym that's crowded with people, past the people who are eating at restaurants inside, maskless. It's just a slap in the face, over and over again. We should not be silencing the voices of healthcare workers. I feel a duty to warn people."[85]

Exhausted and frustrated, healthcare professionals have urged government officials to act, such as a November 24 letter to the Governor of Connecticut from hundreds of physicians, urging him to "halt all unnecessary public gatherings. We are prepared to do whatever we can to care for, comfort, and heal all those that we can, but we want everyone outside to know what we are up against, and not to assume that our capacity is limitless."[86]

---

[84] Fleming N. Coronavirus misinformation, and how scientists can help to fight it. *Nature*. June 17, 2020.
[85] McFarling UL. A "duty to warn": An ER doctor, shaped by war and hardship, chronicles the searing realities of Covid-19. *STAT*. December 21, 2020.
[86] Bernstein L. With hospitals slammed by covid-19, doctors and nurses plead for action by governors. *The Washington Post*. December 3, 2020.

Doctors in Missouri started a petition to push the Governor to issue a state-wide mask order, noting, "We're drowning at the hospital. People are dying every day from covid-19, and we're not doing everything in our power to stop the virus."[87] Dr. Haider Warraich, a cardiologist in Boston, provided these wise thoughts about physicians speaking out, "Social activism is central to the mission of health equity that physicians embark upon the day they first don their white coats. Physicians, nurses, and other healthcare workers are often eyeball to eyeball with the most tragic consequences of societal injustice. Wearing a mask is not a political issue. Racial equity is not a political issue. These matters have been falsely painted as political matters, perhaps to artificially narrow the spectrum of voices that can participate, yet they remain well within the purview of the oath that physicians take."[88]

We also have to be willing to counter the medical misinformation from our colleagues, like Dr. Scott Atlas, Trump's special adviser on coronavirus, who consistently roiled against the CDC's pandemic advice. Healthcare professionals should not be allowed to push bad science and provide bad advice. In my home state of Oregon, a physician and nurse, both outspoken anti-mask supporters, lost their medical licenses for spreading disinformation. Dr. Richard Friedman noted, "As doctors, we are sworn by the Hippocratic oath to do no harm. And there are potentially lethal consequences in telling the public that hydroxychloroquine is a remedy or that face masks don't prevent the spread of infection. Doctors should realize that their advice is, in effect, a form of medicine. If they step outside accepted standards of practice, based on empirical evidence, it's time for the state boards to take disciplinary action and protect the public from these dangerous doctors."[89]

There are some people who are so entrenched in pandemic misinformation and anti-vaccine myths, they are unlikely to listen to reason. Most individuals will listen, provided we also attend to their concerns, as noted by Dr. Dipesh Navsaria, associate professor of pediatrics at the University of Wisconsin School of Medicine, "There's a definite fear that seems to go in two very different directions, I suspect often based around one's political leanings because all this has become politicized. Many are saying I want you to

---

[87] Bernstein L. With hospitals slammed by covid-19, doctors and nurses plead for action by governors. *The Washington Post*. December 3, 2020.

[88] Warraich HJ. Fauci's strategy for effective health advocacy: "You cannot be ideological." *STAT*. July 14, 2020.

[89] Friedman RA. What to do about doctors who push misinformation. *The New York Times*. December 11, 2020.

help me, not to treat me like an idiot or treat me like I'm stupid, I want you to take my concerns seriously—when we take that approach, we're much more successful."[90]

The pandemic is still with us. No vaccine is 100% effective or 100% safe. During the next year we will face renewed concerns about vaccine safety and efficacy. We need to watch and listen, while following safe public health messaging. SARS-2 will not disappear, but we will learn to live with it and manage it, as we do with influenza. Truth in science will lead us out of this pandemic and is our best hope for a healthy and equitable future. The COVID-19 pandemic has reinforced this message, as eloquently noted by Dr. Nicholas Christakis, "A society that feels besieged by the threat of the virus will increasingly treat scientific information, and not just scientists, seriously."[91]

[90] Klass, P. How pediatricians are fending off coronavirus myths. *The New York Times.* November 16, 2020.

[91] Christakis N. *Apollo's Arrow: The Profound and Enduring Impact of Coronavirus on the Way We Live.* New York: Little, Brown, Spark, 2020, p. 368.

Everybody knows that pestilences have a way of recurring in the world; yet somehow we find it hard to believe in ones that crash down on our heads from a blue sky. There have been as many plagues as wars in history; yet always plagues and wars take people equally by surprise.

—Albert Camus, *The Plague* (1947)

Index

For the benefit of digital users, indexed terms that span two pages (e.g., 52–53) may, on occasion, appear on only one of those pages.

Tables and figures are indicated by *t* and *f* following the page number.